3800 04

W9-AAK-462

WITHDRAWN

GETTING TO KNOW YOU

It's a very ancient saying,
But a true and honest thought,
If you become a teacher
By your students you'll be taught.

Getting to know you,
Getting to know all about you…

Anna Leonowens
The King and I

To Maurice and Jean-Pierre

To my students and my patients

And to Pamela

GETTING TO KNOW YOU

A Physician Explains How
Acupuncture
Helps You Be The Best YOU

Joseph M. Helms, M.D.

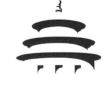

M.A.P.
Medical Acupuncture Publishers
Berkeley, California

First Edition

Copyright © 2007
Joseph M. Helms, M.D., and
Medical Acupuncture Publishers
P.O. Box 815
Berkeley, California 94701-0815

The information and advice in this book are based on the training, professional experience, and research of the author. The author and publisher conscientiously endeavored to ensure treatment descriptions are consistent with the standards of practice generally accepted in the western biomedical and medical acupuncture communities at the time of publication. Any medical indications should not be used as exclusive or definitive recommendations, and should not be the reader's sole source of information nor substitute for professional clinical judgment. Use of medical acupuncture must be done in the context of proper medical care. The author and publisher disclaim any liability, loss, injury, damage, or adverse effects incurred as a consequence, directly or indirectly, of the use and application of any of the contents of this volume.

Library of Congress Cataloging-in-Publication Data

Helms, Joseph M., 1944-
Getting to know you : a physician explains how acupuncture helps you be the best you / Joseph M Helms. – 1st. ed.
    p. cm.
    Summary: "Explains psycho-biological 'types' from the perspective of classical acupuncture texts. Describes the types with patient examples, the experience of acupuncture treatments, and the circulation of acupuncture energy in the body. Recommends self-improvement approaches for likely problems in each type, and gives guidelines for appropriate use of acupuncture therapy for medical concerns"--Provided by publisher.
    ISBN-13: 978-1-57250-712-8 (alk. paper)
1. Acupuncture--Popular works.   2. Self-actualization (Psychology)--Popular works.   I. Title.
RM184.H454 2007
615.8'92--dc22
                    2006032844

Design and illustrations by Glen McKenzie
Front cover photograph by Nyul/Dreamstime
Back cover photograph by Wayne Shimabukuro
Printed in the United States of America

Contents

Also by Joseph M. Helms, M.D.

Acupuncture Energetics
A Clinical Approach for Physicians

INTRODUCTION

This is not a book about needles. Nor is it a book that shows you which acupuncture points to press when you have a headache or a cold or you can't sleep. Rather, it is a book that shows how you can better understand yourself by embracing the time-tested principles of acupuncture. It details the health benefits you can enjoy by anticipating and recognizing the earliest stages of illness. It explains how you can be more thoroughly yourself, and why that's good.

As a young physician I had the good fortune of adding acupuncture to my clinical skills. I say good fortune, because I cannot imagine that I would still be practicing medicine had I not undertaken this additional training. The acupuncture dimension of my interaction with patients allows me to feel like a physician, gives me joy in practicing medicine, and enables me to help my patients in ways that I would otherwise not be able to. Good fortune has followed me through my career. During the past thirty years I have directed a program in medical acupuncture that has trained over five thousand physicians. The passion and commitment that these doctors bring to their revitalized medical practices have allowed acupuncture to enjoy increasing popularity and availability in the United States. This growing public enthusiasm motivated me to organize this material for you.

You can use this book in several ways. The core content revolves around "biopsychotypes," an acupuncture-derived way of looking at our constitutional makeup. This can be a tough concept to grasp the first time through. The material is layered so that each chapter prepares you for the next, and each in turn adds to its predecessor. If you are eager to learn which constitutional qualities are most prominent in your makeup, you may complete the orientation questionnaire in Appendix II and begin with the chapter that describes the biopsychotype associated with your highest score.

If you need to know the role acupuncture might play in a problem you or someone you know is having, you might start by reading Chapter 12 ("What Can Acupuncture Do Best?") and scanning the categories and recommendations in Appendix III. Along the way, you can share the experience of acupuncture treatments and practice by reading the patient and physician quotes at the bottom of the pages.

The stories and quotations are from patients in my practice and students in my courses. They are accurately presented and approved by the people quoted. Several asked that I give them pseudonyms.

In *Getting to Know You* I try to convey the creative intelligence of acupuncture and how it can blend with our western consciousness to enhance our self-knowledge and personal health. I hope you will absorb some of this wisdom of acupuncture and put it to good use for yourself, your family, and your friends. And especially, I hope you have fun and gain insights as you spend time getting to know all about *you*.

Chapter 1
My Story

I am often asked how my interest in acupuncture began, and what happened to sustain my fascination with it for so many years. As many times as I've tried, I have never found a short way of telling the story. Here goes:

Just before I began medical school, in the spring of 1968, I spent some time in Paris. In that season the city was illuminated with burning barricades and passionate public arguments about the future of education, society, and civilization. I had fallen in with a group of French and American graduate students who dissected each day's speeches and events after the demonstrations had died down. During one of these intense late-night dramas, one of my friends, with a theatrical flourish, thrust a book about acupuncture before my eyes. The cover photograph showed a man's face sporting a dozen needles. I had never seen nor imagined such a phenomenon and was astonished by the image and the idea. At the same time, a curious *click* exploded inside me: "Pay attention to this!" I knew something important had just happened, but I didn't know what it was or how central it would become in my life.

That was the moment when the acupuncture seed was planted in my consciousness. I bought the book the next day and read it in a week. (It was the first book I read in French.) I soon discovered that acupuncture was an integral part of everyday medical practice in France and across Europe. I secured introductions to several physicians who practiced acupuncture, and the few hours I spent observing their work stayed in my mind throughout my medical training in California. The fruition and maturation of the acupuncture seed took place during the following dozen years.

I started practicing medicine in 1973, initially in emergency rooms and urgent care clinics and later in my private outpatient practice. Although I had good training and the appropriate diplomas and certificates, much of what brought people to see me had not been covered in classrooms or clinical training. Their complaints seemed legitimate, but

1

they didn't have the full-fledged diseases I'd been taught to diagnose and treat. I knew there was something wrong that deserved attention, and they knew something was amiss. They were recognizing subtle changes in the way they felt, long before the changes could be detected with conventional tests.

I was quietly frustrated during this period. I found little guidance from my textbooks or colleagues about how to deal with these sorts of medical problems. I had no theoretical framework to make sense of the undiagnosed conditions that bothered my patients, and no tools to intervene and change the evolution of their problems. I had not found my place in the profession of medicine.

In 1972 President Nixon traveled to China to meet with Chairman Mao. Press observers accompanying the visit reported remarkable effects achieved by traditional practitioners of acupuncture. One reporter, James Reston of the New York Times, who required an emergency appendectomy during the trip, had all the pain following surgery disappear after needles were placed near his elbows and knees. What was a routine procedure in eastern medicine made headlines in America. In the months following that historic visit, the news media explored acupuncture and other aspects of Chinese traditional medicine and culture. The more reports I read about acupuncture, the more I wanted to learn about it.

I remembered the acupuncture book I had bought in Paris. I was confident – in the same intuitive way as when I first saw the book – that it could contain solutions to my frustration. As I reread the book it became increasingly clear to me that acupuncture offered something that my conventional medical approaches were overlooking. Maybe in the practice of acupuncture there were early treatments for undefined illnesses that had not yet qualified for standard medical diagnoses and treatments. This was my innocent vision as a young physician trying to fulfill my professional ideals. So I went to France in search of acupuncture training.

For three years I shuttled back and forth between California and France, studying in Paris for periods of three weeks to three months and bringing acupuncture books back to Berkeley so that I could continue my studies between visits. During my initial stay in France in 1968, I had learned that acupuncture has been practiced and taught there since the late 1800s. In fact, acupuncture had long been accepted there as a complement to standard medical management, well integrated into the practices of primary care and specialty physicians alike. Acupuncture was in its heyday in France in the 1970s and early 1980s. There were at least ten professional acupuncture societies, four in Paris alone. I admired how these well-trained physicians were incorporating acupuncture into their medical practices and helping patients in ways that they could not have done otherwise.

I was generously received in Paris, both professionally and personally. As I met French physician acupuncturists I was offered many opportunities to spend classroom and clinic time with the best trained and most highly respected practitioners and teachers. The spirit of enthusiasm in their teaching was infectious. There were other foreigners in my group, from Italy, Spain, and Germany, but no other Americans. All doors were open to me, and I was discovering that eastern and western, ancient and modern healing systems – time-tested or double-blinded – not only could be, but had already become quite compatible partners.

As I gained confidence in my acupuncture clinical skills I started treating patients in Berkeley. This was exciting. It was fun. I saw my medical practice evolving, slowly but firmly, into exactly what I wanted it to be. People who did not fit into the standard medical model of sickness and health found that were they taken seriously here, as were people whose problems eluded successful conventional treatment. Together my patients and I found that acupuncture could often bring them relief from their problems.

Learning acupuncture is like learning a new language and becoming familiar with a new culture. At first I saw everything as foreign and difficult, and every step toward expressing myself felt clumsy. Memorizing the points, channels, and funny terms seemed more akin to studying Italian than to mastering a new approach to helping patients. Attaching explanations like "stagnant liver energy" to symptoms of anxiety and irritability or muscle tension seemed far-fetched. In a remarkably short time, however, I grew comfortable identifying and treating explosive headaches as "rising liver fire." I now observe and foster this same acculturation process in the physicians I teach.

The biggest leap I had to make while assimilating the fundamentals of acupuncture was to embrace the notion of "Qi," of acupuncture energy. The quality of Qi in an individual makes the difference between "If all lab values are within normal range, why do I feel the way I do?" in a person with vague but disquieting symptoms, and "I feel great, thanks!" in another patient with equally normal lab test results. I gradually gained a different perspective on energy metabolism and the immune response, which allowed me to understand and treat my tired patients, as well as those with digestive problems, recurring respiratory infections, and menstrual problems. My professors in France had taught me very clearly about the energy disturbances behind muscle tension and joint pain, and these concepts gave me the tools to address the headaches, tight shoulders, backaches, and joint pains my patients came in with.

During one of my seasons in Paris my principal professor, Dr. Maurice Mussat, was meeting several evenings a week with Dr. Jean-Pierre Muyard, a psychiatrist interested in the theoretical foundations of acupuncture. These were not special tutorials aimed at using acupuncture in psychiatry; rather, they were brainstorming sessions exploring correlations between Chinese and western definitions of human psychology. These two physicians were passionately and systematically correlating the concepts of organ functions and influences from the classical texts into contemporary emotional and psychological qualities and abnormalities. The term "biopsychotype" evolved from these meetings, as they redefined and clarified the structural, functional, and psychological attributes of each organ (organ = "bio," emotions = "psycho," hence "biopsychotype"). They developed the constitutional descriptions that I explain in the middle chapters of this book. For me, these meetings were the highlight of that season of training, and the biopsychotypes have been my orientation in acupuncture ever since.

It took me a while to understand the paradigm of biopsychotypes and then to confirm it in my own patients. I started to recognize in my own life and in my practice that our constitutional makeup not only embodies our strengths of physical body and personality, but also creates the likely pattern of breakdown as we encounter the physical and emotional stresses and strains of life. *As we are made up, so do we break down.* Our strongest qualities and characteristics often mirror our weakest links. Equally important, our feeling that something is amiss often reflects early disturbances in an organ's sphere of influence, as defined in the acupuncture texts. The joy for the patient is that his collection of curious observations and complaints can finally make sense to himself and his physician. The joy for the physician is that his acupuncture treatments can restore a healthy energetic balance and physiological function.

As I advanced in my acupuncture training, I saw that my needle patterns could direct the flow of energy through the acupuncture grid of channels and organs. I selected the best points to stimulate by applying the French interpretation of the classical texts. After I grew comfortable integrating the new logic of acupuncture into my practice of medicine, I started needling my patients in Berkeley. I no longer needed to tell them that they would have to "live with it" or refer them to a specialist who would tell them the same thing. I finally felt that I was a doctor equipped to diagnose and treat the patients who sought my services, before they were so ill that they landed in the emergency room.

A year or so after I started seeing patients for acupuncture in Berkeley, I received feedback that confirmed I was on the right path. When she came to see me, **Claudia Jennings** was visiting friends in Berkeley on her way home to London. Her problem was complex, involving insomnia, nasal allergies, bronchitis, digestive difficulties, and protracted menstrual periods. She had been evaluated thoroughly in England in the year prior to this trip, and in the end was told that work and family pressures were at the root of all her problems. Her doctors encouraged her to take the trip that she was now cutting short because her ill health prevented her from continuing.

> *Several doctors told me that I had become a hypochondriac since my divorce. But you convinced me I'm not. I told you what I came to be treated for, and it's a long list. Rather than cutting me short, you asked me even more questions about problems that I had learned not to mention to other doctors, because I had been told that these problems are imaginary or completely unrelated. But honestly, they're not all in my head.*

> *I feel great right now after the treatment. Even if it's months before I have another treatment, I am relieved to know that there is a system of medicine that can link everything that is going wrong with my body and treat it. This whole trip was worth it just to learn that I'm not making things up and I'm not going crazy.*

My vision as a young physician, wanting to thoroughly understand my patients and their problems in order to help them feel better, gradually matured into a vision of wanting to infuse our conventional practice of medicine with the wisdom of acupuncture. Throughout my professional life I have been given opportunities to explore and develop this vision. In 1977 the American Holistic Medical Association invited me to organize an acupuncture course for its physician members. I started with a series of four- and five-day seminars, and by 1980 I had developed a comprehensive training program. The first time I gave the full program there were five participants, but no textbooks or other teaching material in English. A few years later the continuing medical education office at the UCLA School of Medicine began sponsoring the course.

Twenty-five students attended the first program under their auspices. In 1980 I gave up working in emergency rooms, expanded my private practice to combine acupuncture and family medicine, and started teaching regularly.

Momentum in both practice and teaching developed rapidly, far beyond anything I had imagined. My practice was quickly full, and physicians from around the country enrolled in the training courses. Innovative, creative doctors returned time and again, to study and to discuss the many ways they were incorporating this material into their otherwise conventional practices. It has been a privilege for me and my teaching colleagues in the Helms Medical Institute to be intimately involved with so many receptive doctors for such a long time. One of the great unannounced truths about medicine and teaching is that we learn more from our patients and students than we do from our textbooks and professors. During the last thirty years the clinical responses of my patients and the enthusiasm of my students have enabled me to refine my practice and teaching and to continue bringing my vision closer to realization.

I'll offer another patient story, this one about my mother. In 2000 my mother, then ninety-one years old, suffered from low back pain arising from some deteriorating vertebrae and disks. She had always enjoyed excellent health, and this new experience of pain in her body distressed her to the point of mild depression. She went to see her primary care doctor, who sent her to the orthopedic surgeon, who did an MRI and referred her to the spine surgeon in his group. He had scheduled her for surgery to remove a "probable" disk protrusion that was "possibly" causing her pain, when she called to ask for my opinion. I don't have the habit of becoming involved professionally in my family's health issues, so this was an unusual and important event for me. I asked her to postpone the surgery until I evaluated and treated her.

My mother belongs to the generation that follows the doctor's orders without asking about other options. She is also the widow of a physician and had never been at ease with her son's apparent departure from conventional medicine. She very reluctantly agreed to my request. I was surprised at how frail she looked when I saw her, and felt even more strongly that taking her to surgery in this condition was risking her life to treat a problem that was not itself life-threatening. I treated her twice a day for six sessions. With each treatment a bit more of her old vitality returned and another quantum of the pain went away. I arranged for a physical medicine doctor, a graduate of my medical acupuncture training program practicing in my mother's town, to continue the treatments and oversee her physical therapy. She saw him twice a week for a few weeks, then weekly for another month, then monthly for a year. She now has maintenance treatments every three months, and continues to enjoy energetic good health, still free from low back pain.

I tell this story here to demonstrate that, even though most Americans are now familiar and comfortable with the concept of acupuncture, this approach is not commonly sought as the first resort when a problem arises. Too often it is turned to as the last resort, especially by physicians, only after other approaches have failed to help. In my mother's case, the acupuncture treatments not only resolved her back pain and avoided risky surgery, but they also helped her regain her prior clarity and vitality. Acupuncture also saved her medical insurance company an expensive hospitalization, surgery, and rehabilitation.

Reading through the chapters of this book, you will discover that acupuncture can help not only with pain problems, but also with other health challenges that you face. The worldview of acupuncture offers you an understanding and appreciation of your qualities, those that make you who you are and that influence how you work and interact with others. It also enables you to be aware of the disturbances that you are most likely to encounter as you go through life. The wisdom of acupuncture offers a roadmap to understand yourself and recognize the level of manifestation of your troubling symptoms. It can lead you to pursue the common sense approaches that I suggest for each biopsychotype, or to seek professional intervention.

As you absorb the wisdom of acupuncture I hope you understand yourself more fully, and, in the process, appreciate how this model integrates itself into your life and your health care decisions. I want this book to help you in getting to know *you*. My goal is that you will be better able to perceive and evaluate the subtle and not-so-subtle changes in your body, and acknowledge them as normal characteristics, or as early imbalances in your primary constitution, or symptoms of a potentially more serious process. Recognizing a change as an early energetic phenomenon, a musculoskeletal problem, or an established organic disorder allows you to identify your health problems at their level of manifestation. Then you can make intelligent decisions about whether acupuncture or another intervention is indicated to avert a more serious problem.

The practice of acupuncture is thousands of years older than the medicine we have developed in the western world during the past one-hundred-fifty years, yet it holds a vitality and richness that can enhance what is practiced every day by doctors and patients. I would like *Getting to Know You* to foster a lifestyle shift in people who lead a self-examined life. The shift places emphasis on healing and preventing the physical, emotional, and spiritual symptoms and disorders that challenge our lives, as a core necessity to productive and healthy living. The new lifestyle demands a consciousness that detects changes and early signs of illness and treats them at subtle, energetic levels before there is gross involvement of the musculoskeletal system or of vital organs. It demands that you take a greater role in understanding yourself and caring for yourself through your everyday health decisions, as well as in what services you ask of your physician.

GETTING TO KNOW YOU

CHAPTER 2
WHY CAN'T YOU BE MORE LIKE ME?

Five years ago I was examining the rigid neck and shoulders of a new patient named **Renee Carter**. She had been having headaches intermittently for about six months. I recognized immediately that her headaches were coming from the stiff and contracted muscles in her neck and upper back, and I was confident that her problem could respond well to acupuncture treatments. But there were bigger questions: What was causing the muscle tension? Could I help her with that as well?

As I continued my examination I asked:

"Does anyone else in your family have headaches?"

"Yes, my mother sometimes goes to bed with what she calls migraines. I've had a couple like that in my life, but the regular headaches I'm having now didn't start until five or six months ago."

"Were there any changes in your life around that time?"

"Well, I moved in with Jim after we decided to get married. We thought it would be easier to plan the wedding if we were together."

"That's a big change for anyone. Has it worked out well?"

"Yes. We have a great relationship and a lot of fun together. I'm an architect, and he is very supportive of me and my work. Any problems we can usually talk through and come up with a solution. It's his parents that are a pain in the neck. They live nearby and constantly want to help us decide to do things their way."

She hadn't even noticed how she used the phrase "pain in the neck" when talking about his parents. But Jim was in the room with us, and he heard it. Without being asked he started to add his own observations.

I realized soon after entering medicine that a large percentage of the patients I encountered in primary care practice come with problems that are not adequately explained by our biomedical model. Many of them defeat our attempts at categorization with our diagnostic nomenclature and conventional treatment modalities. If a patient has a clinical presentation that cannot be explained or treated by the current

"A month or so after Renee moved in, I became aware that she is quite shy in social settings, almost timid, especially with my parents, but even with small groups of my friends. I had never noticed this about her before, and I figured she just takes a bit longer than I do to get to know people, and that in time the visits would be smoother and more fun. But that's not the case. She disappears behind a screen of polite silence whenever anyone offers suggestions about the wedding. Her sense of humor, her irreverent observations, her generosity...all get lost in this shyness stuff. I don't get it."

"I just don't like all the attention they're giving me and how everyone wants to plan the wedding for us. I'd like for us to do it on our own. I don't want to be rude or ungrateful, but it's our wedding, and they are almost taking over."

"Yeah, you're right. My parents can get pretty pushy. But just tell them to back off. Like I do. Sometimes you have to do that with them."

"But I can't do that."

"Sure you can. I do. Just do it."

*"I **can't**."*

And then, with a combination of exasperation, affection, and gentle bullying, Jim blurted out:

"Why can't you? Just be more like me with my parents. Why can't you be more like me?"

Renee sat silently for a few moments as her face reddened and tears welled:

*"Because I can't. Because I'm not you. Because I'm not like you. I'm **me**."*

---

model, the blame is placed on the patient who does not fit the prevailing view.—*Ivan Iriarte, M.D.*

When I got here, somehow I knew this was the right place. I had already been to the university medical center, and they made me feel like I was just a lamb to the slaughter. I felt you perceived the whole of me, that you saw the many symptoms as making sense. In fact, you elicited these things from me, not just tolerated my tale. I knew on

That was that. She wasn't, she couldn't be, and she shouldn't try to be. Jim was beginning to learn one of the first great lessons of marriage, that the goal is not to mutually mutate into male and female forms of the same being. Rather, the goal is to explore how to live comfortably, productively, and happily with each other's strengths and weaknesses, similarities and differences, and hopefully learn something from each other in the process.

After a little more talking, they both started laughing. They understood how the frustration she had been feeling from his parents' pressures had locked itself into her muscles, and the ensuing muscle tension had started the cycle of headaches. At that point I knew that I could work with both the headaches and Renee's response to Jim's parents, the real triggers of the headaches.

If Renee had appeared during my shift thirty years ago when I was a young physician working in the urgent care clinic, I would have followed the thought process I learned in training: a quick neurological exam to rule out a serious problem within the brain, pain medication for the acute headaches, a trial of the migraine medication of the era, and a referral to the neurologist to rule out any pernicious causes. This is still the approach taken by most primary care physicians today. Not that such a thought process and treatment protocol are inappropriate or wrong, but I think it's at best incomplete and potentially inadequate to identify and address the core driver of problems like Renee's: physical manifestations of emotional stress.

Acupuncture views the human body quite differently from what is taught in medical school. In acupuncture physiology, an organ serves a purpose above and beyond the metabolic functions ascribed to it in western medicine. Each organ generates its own energy and contributes

an intuitive level that acupuncture might be of great value to me.—*Mary Wilson*
Allopathic medicine treats problems people have, while acupuncture treats people with problems. Using acupuncture I really get to know my patients. We become partners in healing, and I share their joy in recovery.—*Marshall Sager, D.O.*
The acupuncture really made a difference in letting me start feeling better physically. For example, I had started physical therapy for my back, but I had given up on

its vitality to maintain the body's structures and regulate its internal balance. When an organ malfunctions, symptoms of imbalance arise. In many cases these symptoms were the very complaints I could not make sense of in the western medical paradigm.

In the tradition of acupuncture, for example, the kidneys not only filter blood and make urine, they also produce energy that influences our body temperature, our bones and bone marrow, our ears and sense of hearing, and the hair on our head. Disorders of kidney vitality can generate not only the gross signs of urinary tract disease, but also subtle symptoms such as internal chilliness, arthritis, hearing loss, and premature graying or hair loss. In acupuncture, each of the body's dozen internal organs has an expanded range of functions for which it is responsible.

Acupuncture reminds us that we each have unique psychological and physical characteristics inherited from our parents. This is the body's constitution that I mentioned in the first chapter. The acupuncture tradition – as interpreted by twentieth-century French physicians – identifies three major constitutional categories called biopsychotypes, each one describing the healthy makeup of a person. This constitutional makeup includes our innate strengths and weaknesses and largely determines our health and illness as we pass through life.

One of the most exciting aspects of acupuncture for me is that what my patients say at our initial meeting takes on meaning well beyond conventional medical interpretations and enriches my understanding of the patient as a whole person. In medical school, we learn to interview patients following a format that starts with the chief complaint, then goes to the background of this problem, and follows with an exploration of the person's past medical history, childhood illnesses, and family

---

it because it wasn't working and it hurt. After two or three acupuncture visits, I went back to physical therapy and was able to move forward with my exercises. After the PT work with deep tissue massage, plus the acupuncture, the soft tissue component of the pain has been minimized. The acupuncture served as the catalyst to move to better responses from other maintenance treatments.—*Thomas Donovan*
The acupuncture treatments have increased my productivity at work. I don't get tired

health patterns. We ask about their social situation and lifestyle habits, and review each organ system with questions to confirm that we have not overlooked any symptoms or information that could be helpful in formulating a diagnosis. This orderly and logical process proves quite useful for a general medical history or an acupuncture evaluation.

With specialization in medicine, however, we risk overlooking features and symptoms of the patients that don't fit into our information categories. We tend to hear only the symptoms and stories that conform to the diagnoses we are considering, and we may dismiss as "irrelevant" the details that arise in the small talk. Striving to arrive at the correct diagnosis of the problem, we often lose sight of the patient. Consider that this challenging intellectual exercise occurs in the midst of a busy practice: It's no wonder that our patients can feel we are neither listening nor hearing.

I believe that my role as a physician is to use my training and experience to help my patients move through their difficulties in life, and to do that I need to understand the how and why of each of their complaints and problems. Acupuncture taught me the value of listening, really listening, to my patients, and helped me to understand what they were saying.

For example, in my early years as a physician, every day patients would tell me:

"I feel tired most of the time."

"I've already had six colds this winter, although I usually don't get more than one. Can you do anything about them?"

"Even though I'm careful about what I eat, my stomach acts up whenever I'm worried about my job."

---

as easy. I can work all day without pain. I can even sit and do paperwork at night for hours. Before I started with the acupuncture I would sit for a half-hour and I'd have to move and stretch until I could sit and relax enough to do some more work. My energy level is up 150% at least. My attitude and my disposition are much more pleasant now because I don't get irritated nearly as quick. My wife notices that I've calmed down and I'm more patient with her, and with the employees.—*Audrose Calhoun*

"My neck and shoulders are always tight by the end of the day."

"I'm often so anxious that I can't enjoy things, but I don't feel right when I take tranquilizers."

"I love salads and I love ice cream, but when I eat either one I feel bloated and very sluggish."

"It's been over a year since the fracture healed, but my arm still bothers me right where it was broken."

"Is there anything you can do about the way I feel before my period? I get really snarly and out of sorts for more than a week."

"What can I do about these headaches other than take more pain pills?"

I spent my time listening to complaints like these, trying to help patients by offering explanations and reassurances. At best, I could alert them to symptoms that, should they occur, might qualify for a "real" diagnosis. At worst, I would prescribe a marginally-indicated drug that briefly made the patient – and me – feel like I was doing something to help. Depending on the day and the setting, between thirty and seventy percent of the patients I saw fit into this category. Listening from an acupuncture perspective completely changed my understanding of people and their problems. It not only taught me how to interpret these questions, but also how to design treatments to help patients with conditions like these.

During my acupuncture studies in France I learned that a disturbance in the *vitality* of a single organ, or a disturbance in the interaction among several organs, can create symptoms that cannot be discovered

I was pretty sick when I first came in here. I used to be an athlete and trained to the point where my body was wiped out. I trained while I had mononucleosis and got really sick. I had to stop swimming. I went from world-class athlete to not being able to walk to class. I even got special license plates to let me park in parking spots for the disabled.— *Katrina Radke*

in their early stages through existing biomedical technology. The same is true with many problems just starting to develop within the organs, problems that are treatable by acupuncture, but are invisible to conventional medicine. Recognized early, these first symptoms can be addressed by psychological and lifestyle changes, diet, acupuncture, or a combination of these personal and professional approaches. But over time, each can develop into a more serious problem, less easily reversible and less easily influenced by acupuncture alone.

Thorough integration of modern acupuncture with western medicine requires an appreciation of the constitutional biopsychotypes, along with their associated strengths and vulnerabilities. Rather than using their Chinese names, I call the three biopsychotypes:

- Vision/Action
- Nurture/Duty
- Will/Spirit

Each biopsychotype represents a duality of positive and negative possibilities, with healthy and less-than-healthy expressions. The qualities and symptoms that identify each biopsychotype derive from the classical Chinese understanding of our makeup, but they are expressed from the perspective of modern western physiology and psychology. Drs. Mussat and Muyard and their colleagues developed this approach during the second half of the twentieth century, and American practitioners have enhanced its value with three decades of clinical experience.

Understanding ourselves and the people we know from the perspective of biopsychotypes helps us to appreciate our own patterns of health and disease. We can identify patterns that link our psychological

---

When I retired I was determined to go fishing the very first day. So I stood there casting all day long, leaning the whole body on one leg with every cast. And that just whacked my spine out of joint. The pain was bad the next day, but I had opera tickets. I had to crawl up the opera house steps to use the side entrance because I couldn't lift my leg without excruciating pain. With that my wife said, "You're going in for acupuncture."—*Bill Kane*

and physical characteristics to the symptoms that bother us. I include this acupuncture dimension in each interview in order to explore more thoroughly who the patient is, what his innate strengths and family health trends are, and in what way he is most likely to become ill. This approach requires that I ask unusual questions, like:

"If I asked you to choose quickly, without really thinking about it, among red, yellow, green, blue, black, and white, which color would you go for?"

"If you had no dietary restrictions and were going to binge on your favorite treat, what flavor would you be looking for: sweet, salty, flavorful or spicy hot, sour-citrus, or bitter?"

These innate preferences help me better understand the person in front of me. I will tell you more about how these questions fit into an acupuncture assessment in the chapters on biopsychotypes.

People usually manifest features of more than one type. Most of us, though, have predominant characteristics arising from one biopsychotype that best explains our main strengths and weaknesses. In the next chapter, we'll explore Renee's problem in the context of her biopsychotype.

I've been HIV-positive since 1983, and was without symptoms for fifteen years. I have a high stress job and was in a destructive relationship. I got stress-related shingles and my T cells dropped. My doctor was alarmed because I had such a virulent case of shingles. He didn't want to treat me further and told me to get my affairs in order. At that time I became more aggressive with antiviral and antibacterial therapy, and I came to you.—
Gregory Marshall

CHAPTER 3

GETTING TO KNOW RENEE

After a few minutes of talking with Renee Carter about her headaches and examining her neck and upper back, I recognized that many features of her constitutional makeup were consistent with the Vision/Action biopsychotype.

How did I know that? First, when she shook my hand, I noticed that her hand was slightly cool and moist, and that she moved her upper body stiffly and turned her head slowly. I also saw some tightness across the middle part of her face, the eyes, cheeks, and jaws—another sign of chronic muscle tightness. Next, her story of muscle tension headaches arising from psychological tension is very typical of Vision/Action people. And finally, her reticence to put herself forward in a social situation, to stand up and be seen and have her opinions heard, is a common quality in one subdivision of the Vision/Action type. I also recognized that Jim and Renee have different constitutional makeups. They are different one from the other, and they were still getting to know themselves and each other.

How does this work? Why do some people have a greater likelihood of holding tension in their necks, while others might have an upset stomach or feel nothing at all? If it's because of our constitutional makeup, is there a way we can change that? Or if we can't change it, can we be less bothered by the breakdown symptoms? To answer these questions thoroughly, let's explore some of the concepts and images used in acupuncture.

Traditional Functions, Traditional Words

Classical acupuncture texts emphasize two important concepts that underlie the model of biopsychotypes:

I had surgery on my back four times. Each time I was fine for a year or two, and then I was just as miserable as before. I really wanted to stop having to take a pill every three or four hours to get through the day. My doctor referred me to you for acupuncture.—*Mary Johnson*
My main complaint of fatigue has been greatly improved by the treatments. My baseline is 85% better than when I started. I still get tired, but can come back now with a

- Each organ has a range of action and sphere of influence that is more comprehensive than that recognized by contemporary medicine.
- The poetic vocabulary of the elements of Wood, Fire, Earth, Metal, and Water is used extensively to describe the behavior of a personality, symptom, or organ.

Organ Spheres of Influence

I already mentioned the importance of the organs' activities in making sense of many common but unacknowledged symptoms. The influence and function attached to each organ allow us to categorize and interpret information about ourselves. Physicians trained in acupuncture use this information to understand what might not be heard by other doctors.

Look at Renee's symptoms: the tendency for her muscles to contract, the headaches she's getting from her tight muscles, sweaty palms, her sensitivity to pressure from forceful personalities, and her profound reluctance to make herself seen or heard, even when her best interests are being violated. From an acupuncture perspective, all these qualities fall under the influence of the Liver, one of the four internal organs whose vitality is manifested in the Vision/Action biopsychotype. We'll look at the other three organs in the next chapter. (I am introducing here the convention of capitalizing the name of an organ when I use it in a traditional acupuncture sense, that is, when it represents its sphere of influence beyond those physiological and pathological qualities typically attributed to it in contemporary western medicine.)

In acupuncture physiology the Liver, in addition to being the metabolic powerhouse described in western medicine, supervises muscles

---

good night's sleep or an afternoon off to read a book. I was starting to get alarmed that I couldn't get my vitality back, and now it is back.—*Mary Ellen Hannibal*
I am struck by the complaints of a chronic nature that I see on a daily basis. I should imagine that these chronic conditions have plagued mankind for centuries, but seem to still evade us in modern medicine. As I studied some of the older traditions in medicine, such as acupuncture and homeopathy, I recognized their applicability for

and tendons and their movement in joints and limbs. It also governs the eyes and vision and, curiously, fingernails and toenails. We saw how Renee's muscles tighten up when she's under stress or when she works at her drafting table. As an architect, she has a refined visual sense, and her mother has talent as a watercolor artist. Renee became nearsighted at puberty and has worn contact lenses since then. Her mother has worn glasses for as long as she can remember and also has concerns about early changes suggestive of macular degeneration. Not all architects and artists come from the Vision/Action constitution, nor do all people who wear glasses, but these factors give us clues which, along with her personality and presenting problems, indicate Renee's constitution.

Five Element Qualities

The second concept from the classical texts is the poetic expression of five elements: Wood, Fire, Earth, Metal, and Water. The words are familiar, but their meaning and value in this context are new. To the ancient Chinese, they represent the fundamental elements of which everything in the universe is composed. They date to the earliest philosophical tradition embodied in classical acupuncture writings. The five elements add an exquisite sense of metaphor and color to acupuncture literature and practice. Each organ is associated with an element. Each element has specific characteristics that distinguish it from the others, such as color, taste, season, and personality. You can find a list of the most important qualities for each element at the beginning of Appendix I.

If you have a strong like or dislike for the color or flavor or season associated with an element, or if you persistently express the psychological traits associated with one of the elements, you may have an early imbalance in the organs associated with that element. Physicians prac-

these and other common problems.—*Donald Counts, M.D.*
One of the problems with our western system is that the right hand often has no idea what the left hand is doing. In my prior practice, my patients would see a specialist for arthritis. The arthritis doctor would give them an arthritis drug. They would see a heart specialist for angina, and that specialist would dispense another drug. I would see them for some gastric upset and, you guessed it, another drug. The interaction

ticing acupuncture routinely use the elemental images in their diagnostic model. For example, the questions about color and flavor I cited
at the end of Chapter 2 derive from the elements. We use the terms and
qualities of the five elements to describe organs, acupuncture channels,
points, functions, personalities, and disorders – the whole spectrum of
acupuncture anatomy, physiology, psychology, and pathology.

Much of Renee's Vision/Action biopsychotype derives from the
Liver attributes and functions that contribute to this type. The old texts
say that Liver manifests the qualities of Wood. Wood, in turn, evokes an
image of a tree, growing upward at the same time as it reaches downward.
A tree is well-rooted and firm, with a sturdy trunk, yet with flexible
branches capable of bending with strong outside forces. In Renee's case,
her healthy Wood qualities have become less flexible than ideal, and, in
fact, the knotty and contracted muscles in her neck and shoulder now
show a Woody texture.

Constitutional Biopsychotypes Revisited

The three biopsychotypes – Vision/Action, Nurture/Duty, and
Will/Spirit – can help us understand how we are constructed, how we
work, and how we break down. All the information included in classical
and modern acupuncture knowledge – the organs' functions, the elements'
influence, and psychoemotional qualities – are coalesced into the biopsychotype descriptive framework. This model thus organizes the multiple
expressions of the human condition, in all its glory and disarray.

Let's explore the components of the term *biopsychotype*, one at a
time. We can start by observing the different kinds of bodies we see.
We need only to go to a public event or shopping mall to recognize the
diversity of body types and shapes. What we don't see is how those

---

of all these drugs, prescribed by caring and well-intentioned physicians, often caused
more problems than the patient had to begin with. I was open to a new approach to
providing health care.—*Marshall Sager, D.O.*
Sometimes it's easy. A patient with a strep throat gets penicillin. A patient with
acute back pain gets some vicodin and a few days off work. The patient may be
happy, but I feel more like a waiter than a doctor. Sometimes it's considerably more

different bodies work inside, what their internal strengths and weaknesses are. This is the *bio* part of the term: the biological functions of the internal organs. We inherit most of our biological aspect from our parents; the rest arises from life's circumstances and the diseases and physical challenges we encounter.

The *psycho* part involves the innate psychological characteristics that contribute to our personality, plus our emotional balance and our responses to internal and external stresses. Together these qualities create biopsychotypes – a descriptive framework for collecting, organizing, and interpreting information about ourselves through meaningful acupuncture associations and patterns. While it's obvious that we inherit some of these psychological qualities from our parents, it sometimes seems the these traits embody the unique strengths and challenges we must develop or overcome as we creatively go through life.

The three biopsychotypes provide an exquisitely valuable organizing matrix both for our self-understanding and for physicians practicing acupuncture. You probably recognize elements of one or both of your parents in your constitutional composition. You have a range of normal qualities, with strengths and weakness in several areas that you share with your ancestors. A review of your family characteristics, illnesses, and behavior patterns can help you predict some of your own strengths and weaknesses.

Your complete constitution probably includes qualities belonging to more than one biopsychotype. But most likely one biopsychotype embodies the bulk of your makeup. Your constitution is composed of strong characteristics along with weak ones. The latter are the seeds of disturbances and deterioration. Throughout life most of us express disorders that arise from imbalances in our dominant biopsychotype.

---

difficult. There are many people whose problems are more complex, people whose complaints do not fit into the precise categories defined in the medical texts. They may be tired all the time, cold, sleepless, suffer from abdominal pain or headaches that have defied diagnosis and resisted treatment. With each successive visit to the doctor they become more frustrated and angry, feeling betrayed by the medical establishment in which they have placed their trust. They had come to believe that physi-

The timing and intensity of the symptoms depend on our core vitality, our age, and the life events that have added to, or detracted from, our inherent resilience.

In the Vision/Action biopsychotype, the most important function of the Liver is to assure the smooth movement of energy and blood throughout the body. This underlies the body's capacity to recover from illnesses, to restore energy, and to move comfortably in both physical and psychological realms. From an acupuncture perspective, Renee has tight muscles coming from an imbalance called "stagnant Liver Qi." This imbalance occurs when the Liver does not adequately promote the smooth movement of energy and blood through the muscles and organs. In Renee's case, prolonged emotional tension initiated the imbalance, although we can assume that, because of her constitutional type, she is more likely than Jim to develop such a pattern. Because stagnant Liver Qi got in the way of adequately nourishing and moistening her muscles, Renee's muscles became painful, tight, and inflamed. And she developed tension headaches.

Qi?

It's pronounced "chee," and you might see it spelled "Chi" or "Ji" or "Ki." Qi is the only foreign word you will read in this book. Often translated simply as "energy," Qi is much more. Qi is the vitality the body derives from its nourishment and circulates to all muscles, organs, and tissues. Moreover, each organ produces its own special Qi that contributes to the overall vitality of the body. More than energy, Qi is the life force that pervades our being, our every thought and action.

Each person's Qi is perceptible, difficult though it may be to describe or define. Qi has to do with the aura of physical vitality and

---

cians, with years of schooling and access to ever-improving technologies, should be able to solve just about any problem. We do the best we can, but commonly it's just not good enough. This is why I turned to acupuncture to broaden my understanding of patients and their problems. I'm sorry they didn't teach me that in medical school.—*Richard Zweig, M.D.*
For me, the turnoff to allopathic medicine came largely from what is imposed: a

the magnetism of personality. It is a quality you radiate, a quality that you can sense in the people you encounter. People possessing exuberant "personality Qi" fill a room the moment they enter, not necessarily by their behavior, but simply by their personal radiance. People who are more contained or introspective may be equally present and active at a gathering, but their presence is not experienced as intensely. One senses the "physical Qi" of a successful body builder differently than someone who simply takes good care of himself. It is easy to discern the difference between the Qi of a hyperactive child and that of a depressed middle-aged businessman, however hard it is to articulate these differences. Qi might be difficult to measure, but you know it's there, in you, and in everyone else.

Students of martial arts cultivate Qi for protection and combat. Consider the movies of Bruce Lee. The rigor of his discipline and the precise application of his mental and physical Qi are evident in his every move. Classes in oriental martial arts are popular throughout the United States. In these classes, students learn about Qi and how to use it for gentle health enhancement or vigorous physical training. They practice the movements in Tai Chi Chuan and Qi Gong to enhance the flow of Qi through the body or to concentrate it in specific areas. Qi Gong masters claim to be able to project their Qi outside their bodies for martial or medical purposes. Yoga studios are common around this country. The postures, movements, and meditations in the yoga disciplines also cultivate Qi, although it's called "prana," for physical health, emotional balance, and mental focus.

A Chinese-American colleague told me how his mother reminisces about the wonderful "kitchen Qi" in her childhood Shanghai home. In fact, his mother asked for her mother's cooking wok as she

---

compartmentalized set of diagnostic codes and permissible complaints and problems. This includes how a patient is allowed to present, how he is supposed to get better, et cetera, et cetera. The other problem is what is ignored or disallowed. The combination of this control over what is allowed and repression of what is disallowed in a simple doctor-patient encounter I feel does violence to the natural presentation of the patient in his dilemma. There is a disconnect and distortion between the patient's

departed for America, because of the good "wok Qi" embedded in it. If we substitute contemporary terms like "spirit" or "energy" or "vibes" for the Qi she describes, we easily understand her. We can comfortably expand the vocabulary of our perception as we sense the Qi in the atmosphere of gardens and buildings and in the vitality radiating from animals and people. Qi is like electricity: We see how it manifests and know how to harness and direct its power, but it is difficult to explain exactly what it is.

Qi permeates all life. It generates warmth in us and stimulates the functions and interactions of the organs. Qi transforms ingested foods, liquids, and inhaled air into blood, fluid, and vitality, and it provides the impulse for respiration, blood circulation, and the movement of fluids throughout the body. Most people are comfortable embracing the idea of a tangible life energy in their physical and psychological makeup. Physicians working effectively with acupuncture in clinical practice must likewise embrace the concept of Qi circulating from organ to organ and throughout the body in precise channels. Over time, we recognize Qi as "real," similar to the way an electrician recognizes electricity as real, in spite of never having seen it.

Before we explore the details of the three biopsychotypes, let's spend some more time with Qi. We'll see a few snapshots of patients and their treatments along the way. You'll get to know these patients better in the biopsychotype chapters and in the quotes that flow along the bottom of each page.

---

experience as reported and the diagnosis and treatment plan. In the orthodox attitude, the implicit definition of quackery or unacceptable professional behavior is valuing the patient's complaint or perception more than the preconceptions of our medical specialty.—*John Giusto, M.D.*
I have practiced emergency medicine for twenty-five years and have seen many changes in therapies and drugs. What has not changed are the patients. They come

CHAPTER 4
MORE ABOUT QI

Snapshots of Three Patients

The acupuncture story begins with Qi. Qi is energy…and much more. Qi flows smoothly from organ to organ through precise, well-described pathways that maintain our vitality. People describe the sensation of Qi being activated during an acupuncture treatment in unique yet similar terms.

Katrina Radke developed chronic fatigue syndrome while training for Olympic competition in swimming. She came for regular acupuncture treatments during her recovery. She says that she likes to feel the energy going through her during the treatment, especially when it's enhanced with electrical stimulation and heat:

> I like to feel it move left to right, down and up, front and back. When I first came in and my head felt thick and swollen from the illness, the needles in my neck and head relieved the pressure and made me feel clearer.

Very aware of her body, Katrina senses the energy movement triggered by the needle patterns, whether clearing her head or *"relaxing the bumps and tensions in my shoulders and lower back."*

In recent years, **Johnny Maddox** has been coming for an acupuncture treatment almost every month to deal with the constant pain and fatigue from spinal stenosis, a problem that makes it difficult for him to walk or move comfortably. He says *"It's like going to the service station for a tune-up."*

He considers acupuncture essential to his life, because it keeps him in control. He can tell the difference in his body and mind if he spaces the

---

in with pretty much the same diseases, the same tales of woe, the same color blood, the same sick organs. I had nothing to offer those who are in chronic pain for whom pain medication no longer works, those who have chronic abdominal complaints and no physical changes, those who have chronic headaches without brain tumor, those who are simply agitated, or depressed, or whose every muscle hurts, or who wheeze, or itch.—*Martha Grout, M.D.*

treatments too far apart. Because Johnny gauges the balance between movement and pain every moment of his day, he is intimately aware of his physical and mental energy – his Qi:

> I know what the results are going to be from a treatment. Twenty-four hours after the treatment there is a snap. It kicks in. It's a sudden load lifted off. A sudden wake-up and I'm no longer feeling heavy and numb. It hits all parts of my body at one time. I get a distance from the pain that gives me the energy and confidence to know I can make it through each day. It's an energy burst in my body, and it lets me feel sharp mentally as well.

Julie Mendosa has always lived her career and home life with exuberance and intensity, but now, in her forties, she can deplete even her abundant Qi. She often arrives at the office with a declaration that "I've spent all my energy. I'm exhausted. Plug me in!" Her response to treatment is another experience of Qi:

> Acupuncture always helps me get my energy back. I'm mellow for a day or two after a treatment; then the energy comes in. It's like finding my center. I feel ten or fifteen years younger for weeks.

Qi and Biopsychotypes

There are three biopsychotypes: Vision/Action, Nurture/Duty, and Will/Spirit. Four organs create the characteristics of a biopsychotype and contribute the energy that flows through its territory of the body. Even before we explore the activities and influences of the organs and how they combine into biopsychotypes, let's look at the energy pathways of each group. Each pair of figures shows one complete subcircuit of energy circulation, with its four organ names attached. In modern acupuncture terminology these organ names are used to identify

---

The acupuncture model takes energetic phenomena into account, along with organic and mechanical problems. Understanding this has allowed me to explain what is happening with patients whose symptoms previously did not make sense. The frequency with which patients present with patterns and disorders that fit the acupuncture conceptualization of biopsychotypes and energy circulation is too great to be explained by chance.— *Ivan Iriarte, M.D.*

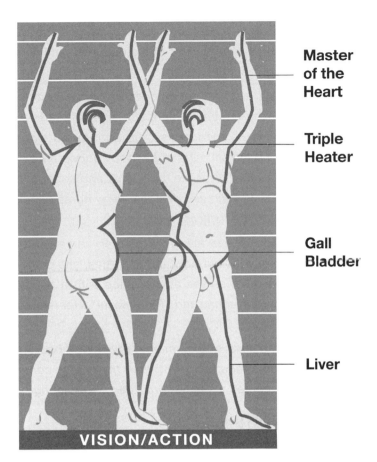

**Master
of the
Heart**

**Triple
Heater**

**Gall
Bladder**

Liver

Figure 4.1   **VISION/ACTION**

the different segments of what is a continuous channel. Each of the energy subcircuits exists symmetrically on left and right sides of the body, like mirror images.

- Vision/Action is composed of energy contributions from Liver, Master of the Heart, Triple Heater, and Gall Bladder (Figure 4.1). The energy channel linked with Vision/Action travels along the

As my own philosophy of health and healing evolved, I sought traditions that respected man as an amalgam of body-mind-spirit, an intricate interlacing of energetic patterns which, at a base, solid, and slower vibrational level materialized into the actual physical beings we are on this earth level. Acupuncture theory and practice has allowed me to understand and manipulate these energetic patterns.—*Terry Bugno, M.D.*

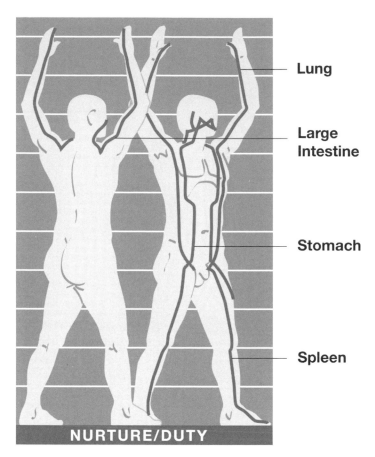

Figure 4.2

side of the head, trunk, and extremities. (Master of the Heart and Triple Heater are the traditional names for the two divisions of the autonomic nervous system. Details are given in Chapter 5.)

- Nurture/Duty is made up of Spleen, Lung, Large Intestine, and Stomach (Figure 4.2). These organs nourish channels that traverse the front of the body.

I am now middle aged, and I'm damned if I'm going to let that beat me down. I don't want to feel at the mercy of the now-vulnerable body, the body that was once invulnerable. I think that my embracing acupuncture and its effects represents a response to those changes. I feel that in middle age I can see things with fewer delusions. I recognize that I'm not invulnerable, I'm not immortal. In acupuncture I never think of myself as a patient. I feel like I'm a partner in this process. I can help the process

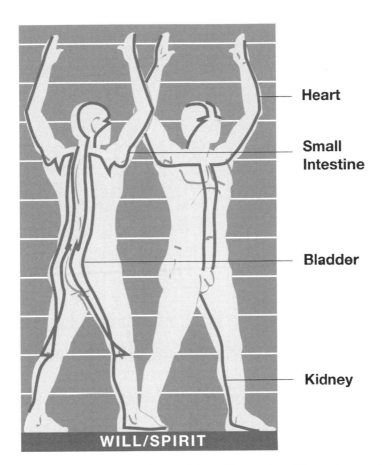

Heart

Small Intestine

Bladder

Kidney

WILL/SPIRIT

Figure 4.3

- Will/Spirit has contributions from Kidney, Heart, Small Intestine, and Bladder (Figure 4.3). Will/Spirit energy runs close to the midline on the front of the body and covers most of the back surface.

Each set of four organs – the energy of one biopsychotype – contributes its constitutional qualities to a person's makeup and supervises the movement of Qi through its region of influence. Each of

along with how I take care of myself, or I could jam it up if I wanted to. It takes a different level of commitment to be an acupuncture patient.—*Joe DiPrisco*
I have sometimes felt that I'm fine and I don't need to come back at six weeks or three months. Then I find myself crashing at four months. Soft signs of impending doom, headaches, non-well-being. I'm able to catch the soft signs earlier on and get in for a treatment.—*Mary Wilson*

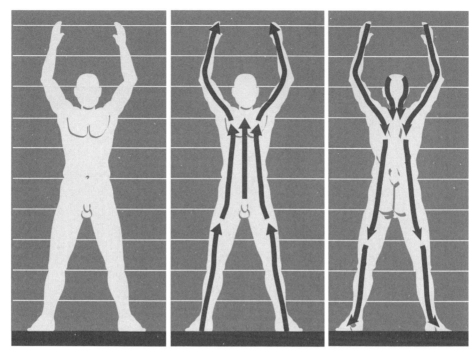

Figure 4.4   Figure 4.5   Figure 4.6

the three biopsychotypes is, therefore, linked to one subcircuit of the acupuncture energy circulation in the body, and each organ and all three subcircuits are indispensable components of a balanced and healthy life. For each of us, however, one biopsychotype – one division of the energy grid – stands out in our constitution.

The Circulation of Qi

Qi flows through major channels in the muscles and through tributaries of the major channels out to the surface of the skin and deep to the internal organs. The pathways these channels follow have

The thing I noticed first when I left was that my mind was clear. I was less stressed, more relaxed. Usually acupuncture helped me read and focus, but sometimes the treatments made me tired and I had to sleep. Sometimes the benefits lasted three days, but then I'd overwork or overstudy. Now treatments last four to six weeks.—*Katrina Radke* Although I came in for my upper back, I think the best benefit I've gotten from the acupuncture is a sense of general physical and psychological well-being. My mood

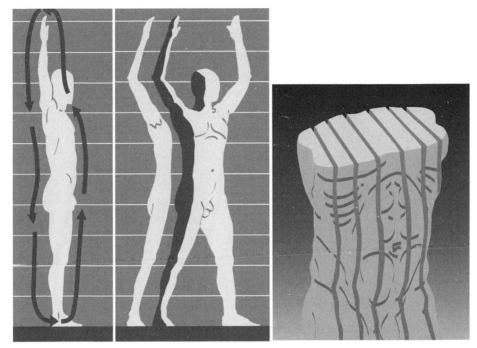

| *Figure 4.7* | *Figure 4.8* | *Figure 4.9* |

been consistent in illustrations throughout the two thousand years of acupuncture's documented history. The "natural" anatomical position in acupuncture shows the human body with the arms raised above the head and the palms facing forward, representing man living in dynamic balance between the Qi of heaven and the Qi of earth (Figure 4.4). Qi flows from bottom to top in the channels on the front of the body, from feet to upraised hands, from earth to heaven (Figure 4.5). On the back of the body, Qi flows from top to bottom, from heaven to earth, thus completing a continuous circuit (Figure 4.6).

---

has been stable, and for two or three days after the treatment my libido was increased. It had been dropping because of the pain in general. I have more energy to do things longer during the day, and more energy to begin projects and whatever needs to be done. I don't get tired as quickly when I start something new.—*Thomas Donovan*
Just picture being up all night with a patient with emphysema who is struggling to breathe. You took care of him last month with the same problem. After he left the hospi-

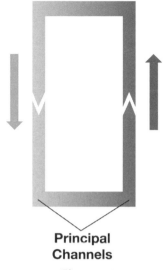

Principal Channels

Figure 4.10

The classical Qi pathways define three pairs of energy circulation subcircuits, which are created by couplets of front and back channels connected at the extremities (Figure 4.7). Each subcircuit influences the section of the body's skin, the muscles, and the four organs through which it flows (Figures 4.8). This network of major channels is the same on both left and right sides of the body, shown conceptually in Figure 4.9. These channels are the "principal channels" or "principal meridians" and are considered to be the interstate highways of the acupuncture roadmap. One principal channel subcircuit is represented schematically in Figure 4.10, with upgoing energy shown on the right side of the drawing, and the downgoing on the left.

In California, Interstate Highway 5 connects the cities in the south with those in the north. It is our principal south-north circulation channel. It flows without interruption between San Diego in the south and Redding in the north and flows through Los Angeles and Sacramento, two of the major "organs" of the California body. If a car stalls in the center lane of a major highway during morning rush hour, traffic coming from residential regions will be slowed or stopped on its way to the city's business center. Circulation in Los Angeles can be influenced by a traffic jam halfway between San Diego and Los Angeles. Once the stalled car is removed, traffic can flow smoothly again. Similarly, blockages in the main Qi highways in the body can cause malfunction or pain. Inserting acupuncture needles at the right junctures unblocks the

tal, on oxygen, he continued to smoke and developed a new pneumonia. This is the kind of inefficient, wheel-spinning treatment process that is disillusioning and discouraging to young doctors. Confronted by this level of dissatisfaction as a resident, I looked at a variety of holistic and alternative approaches. Stress management, acupuncture, herbs, and other natural approaches always made more sense to me than much of the after-the-fact medicine we practice in the academic centers.—*Victor Sierpina, M.D.*

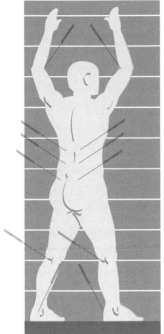

Figure 4.11

congested energy flow and allows the movement to balance itself, thus correcting the malfunction or relieving the pain.

An acupuncture treatment pattern typically involves needles in the leg and arm sections of the front and back channels, which, working together, will push energy into circulation up the front and into the organs, and then pull energy from the upper part of the body through the muscles and back down to the lower part. The needles in the extremities of the channels are like feeder lights and highway patrol officers directing the volume and speed of traffic moving into the main circulation route once the obstruction has been removed.

Johnny Maddox has chronic pain in his lower back where the nerves and muscles are most affected by the spinal stenosis. Because the energy flow gets jammed up in that region, I always insert needles deeply into the lumbar muscles. I also use heat and electrical stimulation to further encourage the flow of energy through the area and to reprogram the nerve firing patterns that carry the pain signals to his brain. In addition to the local needles for his pain, I insert a pattern of needles in his legs and arms to push the Qi through the channels flowing through this painful region (Figure 4.11). In the traffic flow metaphor, his back pain is equivalent to a ten-car pileup behind an overturned tractor-trailer, backing up traffic for miles. The needles in his lumbar region are the tow trucks that clear the damaged vehicles and restore the flow of traffic.

My interaction with my regular doctors is a disconnection between who I am, what I feel, and my body. My internist is never really looking at me; he is sending me to get blood tests. When I tell him what is going on, he has a good reply to show he is keeping up with the journals, but it is more theoretical and detached, and it doesn't feel like he relates to me. I am grateful for western medicine and what it can do, but I've never had any other kind of transaction than this. Acupuncture is more about

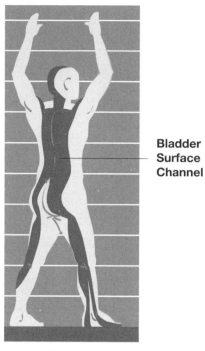

Bladder
Surface
Channel

Figure 4.12

The Tributaries of Qi

Surface Channels

Specific needle patterns can also provide access to other levels of energy circulation. For example, needling points at one end of a principal channel—alongside the toenails or fingernails—activates a special "surface channel" that travels through the outermost layers of the body, like a broad energy band overlying the pathway of that principal channel (Figure 4.12). The network of surface channels in the skin and subcutaneous tissues creates a protective energy field that surrounds the body and buffers it from the extremes of heat, cold, damp, dryness, and wind. The energy that circulates in these surface pathways serves as a barrier that shields the internal organs from external living and working conditions. This protective Qi functions as a sort of acupuncture immune system, an energetic first response to trauma and external conditions. The surface channels and their relationship to the principal channels are represented schematically in Figure 4.13.

One day **Bill Kane** came to my office on short notice because he had strained his back while gardening the previous day. He had pain from muscle spasm in his right lower back that worsened when he tried to straighten up

healing and less about getting rid of symptoms, although it does that too.—*Mary Ellen Hannibal*

What was utterly fascinating to me was that while I was going through this educational process I was getting information that began to put all of medicine together for me as far as understanding patient problems and how these problems evolved. It was as if in medical school we all learned the pieces of a vast puzzle to the point that

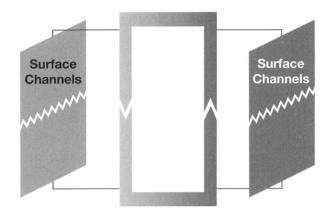

Figure 4.13

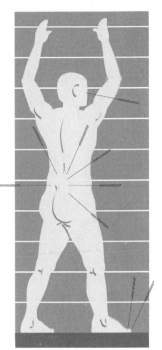

Figure 4.14

to walk. I examined the area of the spasm and identified the two principal acupuncture channels that travel through that region. To activate their surface pathways, I would need needle points beside the right fourth and fifth toenails, where those principal channels end.

Bill doesn't like having needles put into the toes—no one does. I convinced him that the treatment is very effective, so he figured it was worth tolerating the insertion discomfort and accepted those needles. Fortunately, his pain and spasm were limited to one side of the back, so I only needed to treat one foot. I had Bill cough while I inserted needes into the two toes. This distracted his attention just enough for him to ignore the initial discomfort. With the activating needles for each of the surface channels in place, I next inserted a needle into the right side of his face to pull the energy of the two surface channels toward it (Figure 4.14). Finally, I placed a half-dozen needles fairly superficially—about one-quarter

we could take the pieces and break them up into smaller and smaller pieces. But we learned nothing about putting the puzzle together, and it wasn't until I was in the acupuncture training program that medicine began to make true sense to me.—*Lowell Kobrin, M.D., Ph.D.*

My patients feel that I care about them more because I am willing to try something like acupuncture. Acupuncture helped me understand that the signs and symptoms

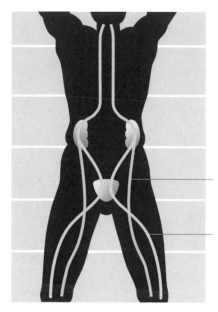

Kidney Organ Channel

Bladder Organ Channel

Figure 4.15

to one-half inch deep—into the flesh overlying the pain and tight muscles in his back. These were the local focusing needles, inserted to draw the attention of the energy movement to the zone of obstructed energy flow.

A circle of redness formed on the skin around the local needles, indicating that the excess energy blocked up at the tight spastic spot was being moved and released and that the heat and inflammation and pain were dissipating. Indeed, after a half-hour of treatment, the redness blanched and I removed the needles. Bill was immediately able to stand upright and rotate at his waist without pain. He phoned the next day to announce that he had slept well and was going to play a gentle game of tennis that afternoon.

Organ Channels

Exits from California Highway 5 take traffic into large metropolitan areas. The carpool high-occupancy vehicle lanes that allow drivers to proceed from the interstate highway directly into the city center, bypassing the toll booths and slow traffic, mirror the "organ channels" in the acupuncture energy circulation network. These channels exit from the principal channels at the large joints—knees, hips, shoulders—and go

the patients present with are very important and need to be addressed in the treatment, even prior to our labeling them as a particular disease.—*Todd Lininger, M.D.*
Now I have an entire world of pathophysiology that explains things to me and to the patients so we can begin to intervene effectively. Acupuncture has taught me patience. I understand the time lines of illness, the root and branches of illness, a unifying theory for someone's eighty-five different complaints. Sometimes I am ahead of them and go

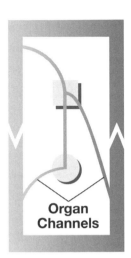

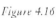

Organ Channels

Figure 4.16

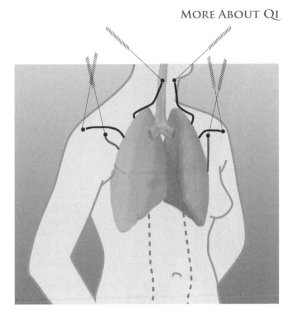

Figure 4.17

deep, directly to the affiliated organs (Figures 4.15 and 4.16). The organ channels provide the acupuncturist direct access to the metabolic activities of an organ. Acupuncturists reserve these channels for problems that involve the organs themselves, such as obstruction, inflammation, or metabolic malfunction.

A few years ago **Mary Wilson** arrived for a three-month follow-up appointment in early December with only a mild respiratory infection, having successfully survived the autumn, the season in which she is most vulnerable to lung problems. The infection did not require antibiotics, but had evolved into a bothersome laryngitis. Mary feared the laryngitis would prevent her from singing in the Christmas chorale, an activity she loves. Her treatment involved a needle pattern to stimulate the Lung organ channel, which passes through the lungs, the vocal cords, and throat, plus additional focusing points for her laryngitis (Figure 4.17). I inserted needles at the top

---

through their biopsychotype and ask them other things that they may be prone to, and they are amazed and imagine that I am wise or psychic. And all I'm doing is listening to them.—
Noel Nowicki, M.D.
I feel from talking with my colleagues that the huge amount of emotional energy that goes into controlling patients, rather than interacting with them for consensual decision-making, is a major contributor to stress and burnout among physicians. Many

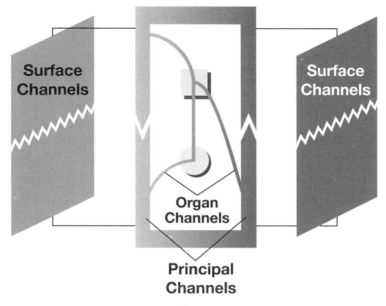

Figure 4.18

of her chest and in her neck and connected them to an electrical stimulator, expecting that this would help break up and move the phlegm and diminish the swelling contributing to her laryngitis.

I left the needles in place for fifteen minutes with the electricity buzzing. Mary rested her body and her voice that day. By the next day, she was feeling back to full strength, well enough to participate at half-voice in the rehearsal for her performance. Three days after the treatment she sang comfortably for the two-hour Christmas concert.

Mobilizing Qi

The different layers of the Qi network are intimately interconnected, and are illustrated schematically in Figure 4.18. Understanding

never learn the value of shooting the breeze with patients, and they feel obligated to deliver more decisions per minute than a district court judge in Calcutta. Gradually they come to hate the intensity of the patient contact. Physicians using the expanded acupuncture paradigm quickly realize that the very process of going deeply into the history, accepting the reality of the patient's symptoms, can often lead to an innovative and gratifying therapeutic approach. Sometimes, in some mysterious way, some

the subcircuits and the tributaries of this network is critical to planning an effective acupuncture treatment. Physician acupuncturists must identify the location, nature, and depth of manifestation of a problem and ascertain whether it is early or chronic, functional or organic. We do this by interpreting as much information as we can elicit from our patients, as well as by employing all the diagnostic tools and techniques of conventional medicine. We then select the acupuncture subcircuit or tributary that will best treat the problem. Through surface channels we can relieve recent pains, but not more chronic pain problems. With principal channels, we can move energy through regions of chronic musculoskeletal pain, but we must use the deeper organ channels for chronic organ problems.

Planning the acupuncture treatment involves linking the most important symptoms to their responsible organs and channels. The goal of the treatment is to restore the organs to their former fully functional state and to reestablish the balance of energy that defines good health. We select for our attention the subcircuit of the neediest organs (unless the problem is on the surface of the body or restricted to one organ, in which case we would select the appropriate surface or organ channel). We arrange the needle pattern in the malfunctioning subcircuit and stimulate strong energy-moving points on the arms and legs to increase the flow of Qi through the entire subcircuit.

Points on the torso and local points overlying a painful region focus the channel flow to the organ or to the area needing attention. The increased flow of Qi allows the body to direct and use what energy it needs for repair and healing. Understanding how to stimulate the energy circulation network gives us the flexibility to influence many medical

form of cortex-to-cortex healing begins to take place, and that catalyzes the healing process.—*Patrick Magovern, M.B.B.S.*
Although I was pleased with what I learned as an acupuncture student, I was startled at the results I obtained as an acupuncture patient. The beneficial effect started even during the lengthy interview. There was so much genuine interest and caring about me and my medical practice that I noticed my own psychology shifting to a more

disorders by moving Qi, and to use acupuncture either as the exclusive treatment or as a complement to other approaches. This ancient medical art is remarkably adaptable to modern medical practice.

How do we know we're needling the right spots? We insert needles to a depth where the patient and the acupuncturist experience a curious sensation. The patient feels a dull, heavy, aching sensation, quite different from the prick of the needle piercing the skin as it first enters the body. The acupuncturist feels the flesh resist the turning or advancing of the needle, and the muscle gives the impression that it is grabbing the needle. With the arrival of this sensation, we know that we have contacted the Qi of the channel and the organ. By activating the entire subcircuit with the needle pattern—plus turning the needles, heating them, or stimulating them with electricity—we add more energy from outside the patient into his circulation. The added energy and stimulation help to move the Qi through the subcircuit and, ultimately, to build up the resilience and reserves of the body.

Mary Wilson declares that:

The needles are not as invasive as pills. The energy from the acupuncture treatment allows me to take charge and shift the responsibility for my respiratory health from the drugs to my own body. The needles make me feel like my body can cope with my illnesses, and I like the idea of enhancing my body's own vitality instead of compromising its response through drugs.

I especially like the declaration from **Joan Kip**:

Acupuncture brings me back to my Self! For me, this is the prime reason I come for acupuncture. My bones ache less, my health improves, but all that follows from getting back to Me.

---

receptive state for the placement of needles.—*Dominick Bachowski, M.D.*
Making a connection with my body and the person who is assisting me with it is very important. Listening to me, seeing me, what I say, seeing through your own eyes, makes a huge difference. It makes the idea of coming for medical acupuncture more attractive than going to the internist. I'll see a conventional practitioner if I have an acute symptom that I can't stand living with, because he will put it under

Many patients express their experience under the needles less eloquently than those I've quoted here. They commonly use such general terms as "relaxing," "refreshing," "restoring," and "energizing." And patients vary in how long the effects of enhancing and moving Qi endure. It might be several days, several weeks, or several months. The duration of a change reflects the complexity of the problem and the amount and quality of Qi accessible within a given patient.

Qi is the essence of life and all of life's activities. Tapping into the wisdom of acupuncture means understanding the importance of Qi as it circulates through our bodies and as its qualities are allocated to the organs and channels. In the next three chapters I present the characteristics of the three constitutional biopsychotypes. By comparing your own qualities to those described, you will gradually get to know yourself, your family, and your friends in this new context. More importantly, you will learn to recognize early changes that allow you to address an emerging imbalance before it becomes too difficult to correct.

---

control. But I know that I am not being healed from that. I will see an acupuncturist for no matter what goes on, acute or chronic, just to get my body going. I love acupuncture. It makes total sense to me. I have a keen perception of the differences among mind and emotion and body in me, and have the intuitive knowledge that they are connected. Acupuncture helps integrate those connections.— *Mary Ellen Hannibal*

I emerged from an uneventful conventional background of surgery, anesthesiology, and pain management. When I entered practice, it soon became obvious that the system I was trained in was completely inadequate in caring for many of the patients I was seeing.—*Todd Lininger, M.D.*

At first I saw acupuncture as another skill to help my patients in chronic pain, but I soon discovered that it is much more than that. It is a way out of the sorry, deperson-

CHAPTER 5

VISION/ACTION BIOPSYCHOTYPE

Social shyness, reluctance to speak out, sensitivity to pressures from other people, nearsightedness, tight neck and shoulder muscles, and headaches that run in the family – these are some of the features in Renee's makeup and symptoms that place her squarely in Vision/Action terrain. But not everyone of a Vision/Action constitution will have all of Renee's qualities or difficulties. Her characteristics are associated primarily with the Liver sphere of influence and Wood elemental features of Vision/Action. But each biopsychotype embodies the functions of two elements and four organs. Stagnant Qi, anxiety, and tight muscles, however, are characteristics common to almost all manifestations of Vision/Action.

Between Psyche and Soma

The interaction between psyche and soma, between our emotions and our bodies, finds expression in the organs and functions of the Vision/Action biopsychotype. How well balanced we are in our emotional and physical lives reflects how this constitutional division is executing its specific responsibilities. The Liver, the Gall Bladder, and the autonomic nervous system (ANS) are the organs and functions associated with the Vision/Action biopsychotype. Most people living and working in our modern society experience some disturbances in the Vision/Action sphere. You'll certainly find some of yourself in this chapter, possibly quite a bit.

The Vision/Action Biopsychotype

If the predominant biopsychotype in your constitution is Vision/Action, you are generally comfortable making decisions and planning.

---

alized, mechanized state of modern medicine, and a way back to the ideal: where the doctor can sit, listen, and touch his patient, and the patient, being heard and touched, can feel the comfort a doctor can provide.—*Richard Zweig, M.D.*
I know that most patients, given the option, would prefer to be under the care of a physician trained in acupuncture rather than a nonphysician acupuncturist. This is simply because of our ability to integrate allopathic and acupuncture approaches and

You are usually full of movement and projects, can be muscular in build and agile in sports, and are blessed with good energy and good digestion. Warm and spirited, you are confident that everything will work out. Your innate talents can be visual or manual. You are independent, courageous, and loyal.

At the active end of this constitution's spectrum, people with a predominance of the Vision/Action biopsychotype in their makeup can be highly motivated and always on the move: putting their projects in place, pursuing sports for the love of activity, competing for the joy of moving. At the quiet end of the spectrum, they can use their creative intellects and visual talents to resolve organizational problems or to design exceptionally functional living and working spaces. They are reluctant leaders, not because they shirk responsibility, but because they prefer to work independently or in a team as an equal player, and do not like to be in the forefront.

Functions and Influences of the Vision/Action Organs

In the acupuncture model of health, Liver and Gall Bladder vitality allows us to make decisions, initiate activity, complete projects, and adapt to life's challenges with flexibility and creativity. Wood is the elemental quality attached to Liver and Gall Bladder energy.

Wood is metaphorically best represented by the image of a tree, a living entity that, like human beings, is balanced between dynamic forces as it goes through life's activities. A tree embodies the life cycle in its ability to awaken with vitalizing sap in springtime, to blossom and bear fruit, and to change color and drop leaves before becoming dormant in

---

make appropriate treatment decisions and referrals if a problem is more dense than acupuncture alone can handle.—*Lowell Kobrin, M.D., Ph.D.*
A good friend referred me to a different acupuncturist. But I wouldn't go see him because he is not a physician. I would not have felt comfortable seeing someone who would treat without understanding western physiology, biomechanics, and pharmaceuticals.—*Joe DiPrisco*

winter. Wood is the only living element in our collection. As such, it is a symbol of the power to come alive, to be infused with energy, and to deal with to the changes imposed by life.

The Wood qualities of this biopsychotype help our bodies and psyches accommodate to the physical and emotional stresses we must endure. Thus, the energy of Vision/Action is indispensable for maintaining physical and emotional well-being.

Katrina Radke embodies mostly Wood qualities. She was a swimmer in Olympic training until chronic fatigue syndrome forced her to stop. Her body is strong, sinewy, flexible, and energetic, and her personality is vivacious. Chronic fatigue forced dramatic changes in her lifestyle, but she adapted creatively and successfully to them by carefully nursing herself while in graduate school studying clinical psychology. Since graduation she has combined her competition sports experience, professional training, and Vision/Action motivation in her jobs, first as a pharmaceutical representative, and then as a facilitator of an initial public offering. Currently she is a university swim team coach.

The autonomic nervous system, the other "organ" associated with Vision/Action, quietly maintains and regulates the essential but usually unrecognized activities of blood circulation, body temperature, transit of food through the digestive tract, and absorption and distribution of fluid in the body. The traditional acupuncture names for these functions are the "Master of the Heart" and the "Triple Heater." The combined functions of Master of the Heart and Triple Heater, in effect, encompass the contemporary physiologic responsibilities of the autonomic nervous system, the unsung hero of internal movement, metabolism, regulation, and homeostasis.

The acupuncturist must do his job right. But in order to put the patient at ease there is an interchange, humor, laughter, an emotional component that transcends the clinical professionalism. The doctor needs to be able to put the patient at ease and to take control, while being very conscious of the person's mental state at the time. Humor can neutralize the situation and diminish any discomfort during the treatment. Humor keeps me alive. If I can't find humor in facing a life-threatening illness

Master of the Heart directs the Heart in its function of pumping blood through the lungs, brain, and all the tissues of the body. (Master of the Heart is referred to variously in translations as "Heart Protector" or even "Pericardium." Its Chinese character is a hand enclosing and protecting the Heart.) The Triple Heater oversees the production and distribution of energy in the body, the nourishing, moistening, cooling, warming, and movement necessary to maintain life energy. Triple Heater represents the body's three cavities – chest, abdomen, and pelvis – in which the digestion, absorption, assimilation, and excretion of ingested liquids and foods take place.

Master of the Heart and Triple Heater are associated with the elemental qualities of Fire (as is the Heart that they protect). The image of *Fire* embodies the sun and illumination, vitality and warmth, rising energy, excitement, and mental brilliance. Fire implies heating and circulating, physical and emotional warmth, enthusiasm, and passion. Qualities of both Wood and Fire are present in the characteristics, influences, functions, and disturbances of the Vision/Action biopsychotype.

These all sound pretty good as core characteristics of a biopsychotype. So how is it that disturbances in this sphere commonly cause our emotions to wreak havoc in our muscles or our digestive tracts? The answer goes back to the traditional influences and functions of the Liver and autonomic nervous system. Each organ's functions are important in the overall energetic balance of the body, but those of the Liver are most vital to maintaining a harmonious interaction between our internal and external states.

---

or pain, then I am going to live a miserable life.—*Gregory Marshall*
My life as a physician has been made hugely more meaningful, enjoyable, and sat-isfying by my study of acupuncture. Learning acupuncture led me to study nutri-tion, homeopathy, and environmental medicine, and as a result my diagnostic and therapeutic paradigms have been expanded. I have realized that most patients with difficult-to-treat disorders are not neurotic. Medicine has just not caught up with

Functions and Exaggerations of the Liver

In Chinese medicine, Liver influences muscles and tendons, the eyes and vision, and fingernails and toenails. Liver and Wood are associated with the season of spring, light blue, blue-green, or green colors, and sour or citrus flavors. When analyzing Renee Carter's presentation, I stated that the most important function of the Liver is to assure the smooth movement of Qi throughout the body. By nourishing the skin and muscles with Qi, the Liver enhances the body's resistance to potentially harmful external conditions and allows it to recover from injuries. Further, the Liver regulates the quantity of blood and body fluids in the circulation through release during activity and storage during rest, thereby assisting the body's daily capacity to recover and restore energy. The Liver influences ligaments, tendons, and muscles, the tissues responsible for movement. A healthy Liver allows flexible joints and good muscle action, along with good nails and good vision.

In acupuncture physiology, the Liver does more than move energy and blood smoothly to organs and muscles and skin. It also enables a strong spirit and drive to express itself through clear planning and direction. The vision that Liver supervises is not limited to what we see with our eyes; it also involves the clear sight of creativity and confident self-expression. The role of the Liver in the body's energetic ecology resembles that of a military general responsible for the overall planning and execution of a military campaign. If our Liver is functioning well and our Qi is flowing smoothly, our personality will be easy-going and happy with freely expressed emotions. If it is not functioning well, our emotions are likely to manifest less smoothly somewhere within Liver's sphere of influence.

---

them.—*Patrick Magovern, M.B.B.S.*
One benefit of doing acupuncture is that my patients who use other complementary therapies have come out of the closet about them. They were afraid to discuss them with other doctors for fear of ridicule. They concluded, rightly, that since I did acupuncture I would be more open to discussing and using other approaches as well.—*Victor Sierpina, M.D.*

The disturbance pattern called "stagnant Liver Qi" occurs when the Liver does not adequately promote the smooth movement of Qi and blood. We saw this in Renee's muscle tension headaches. Emotional tension, if intense and prolonged, can initiate or aggravate stagnant Liver Qi in our physical bodies. Reciprocally, stagnant Liver Qi can produce or exaggerate emotional agitation. We can experience stagnant Liver Qi at one or multiple points along a physical-to-emotional spectrum of symptoms. Physically our muscles may feel stiff or contracted when we move because the Qi and blood are not moistening and nourishing adequately. Muscles may become painful or inflamed, even to the point of tension in the jaw, eyelid spasm, or a facial tic. The emotions of frustration, impatience, irritability, and resentment emerge when Liver Qi is obstructed. The dynamics act in both directions: emotional tension can be both the effect and the cause of stagnant Liver Qi.

Fight-or-Flight, Restore-and-Relax

The autonomic nervous system (ANS, the combined Master of the Heart and Triple Heater) is an important part of Vision/Action influence. When working properly, it keeps our important internal activities moving smoothly and in balance. The ANS is the division of the nervous system that most quickly manifests emotional distress or well-being. This is our fight-or-flight and restore-and-relax mechanism. It makes our hearts beat fast when we are chased by angry dogs or slow down when we are deeply relaxed. In response to our work or home environment, our autonomic system can be set too high and be overly reactive to physical and emotional stimuli. Or it can be set too low and become exhausted, and we may be aware that everything inside us moves slowly. The symptoms generated by an off-kilter autonomic

---

For those patients with fatigue and normal labs that I never had anything to offer, I now have some new tools in my doctor's bag. Everyone instinctively believes that anger, fear, depression, and overworking can cause illness, so it's nice to have a system that automatically incorporates these factors into a syndrome instead of searching whether the illness is organic or psychosomatic.—*Norman Solomon, M.D.*
Training physicians in medical acupuncture will have a powerful influence on the

nervous system are remarkably varied, from being intensely aware of every heartbeat to having a vague sensation of low energy or sluggish digestion.

It is the autonomic nervous system that brings Fire qualities to the Vision/Action biopsychotype. Fire connotes summer, the color red, and bitter or burned flavors, and is associated with the Vision/Action functions of Master of the Heart and Triple Heater.

Stagnation of the Liver moving Qi through the body, a Fiery state in the emotions, or a change in the functions of the Vision/Action organs can affect your personality, your vision, neck muscles, heart, or digestive system. Stagnant Liver Qi creates physical symptoms that are unique for each person; the range of possibilities is immense. When this division is out of balance, however, there is always frustration or anxiety.

The characteristics and symptoms cited in this chapter can occur in almost any combination, in people of any biopsychotype. An individual's genetic constitution and psychological balance determine whether a disturbance remains as a manageable habit or personality trait, or evolves into a bothersome physical or psychological symptom. The intensity of expression is also influenced by the individual's other strengths and weaknesses that might soothe or inflame the disturbance. Four common patterns occur in Vision/Action people.

Four Common Patterns of Disturbed Liver Qi

Fidgeting

A person with predominant Liver and Wood qualities might express the early presence of stagnant Liver Qi by tapping his fingers or foot, clicking his pen, or getting up and pacing. These behaviors are

---

direction of medicine. Physicians practicing acupuncture have new tools that complement those of conventional medicine. Understanding acupuncture allows us as physicians to appreciate the unity of body, mind, and spirit, and to appreciate the subtlety of the human form. Acupuncture shows us how we can intervene to promote wellness as well as treat disease, and encourages us to be humble in the face of twenty-five hundred years of clinical experience.—*Mitchell Elkiss, D.O.*

expressions of frustration or anxiety, stagnant Qi trying to move. He knows that if he can run or pick up a basketball game later in the day that most of this tension will be discharged. In fact, he *must* exercise regularly and vigorously to maintain his sense of balance and well-being. Not to exercise increases the fidgeting and can lead to holding tension in the upper back and neck muscles. The tension and impatience cause sudden eruptions of irritation in an otherwise easy-going personality. This person is likely to have his own unique sense of physical order, invisible to those around him. Disturbing his order risks injury to the relationship with the disturber.

You certainly have lived with or worked with someone like this, or you might have these habits in your own makeup. One of the most common expressions of disturbed Liver Qi, this disharmony can usually be brought back into balance through increasing exercise and limiting autonomic nervous system irritants, such as caffeine and alcohol. These symptoms are unlikely on their own to bring a person to acupuncture for help, but they quite commonly accompany more serious complaints.

Impatience and Tight Muscles

Someone of similar constitution but more on the quiet end of the spectrum might habitually doodle on scraps of paper while talking on the telephone. In those who have not yet discovered the importance of exercise or who cannot include enough movement in their daily lives, stagnant Qi can lead to increasing impatience and irritability in their personalities and to chronic muscle tension patterns in the upper back, sides and back of the neck, or jaw. These people can be seen frequently rolling and twisting their heads and kneading their necks and shoulders. More advanced states include a silent but chronic criticism of others

---

I decided to take the acupuncture course after three patients in one day asked for a referral to an acupuncturist. Surprisingly, at least to me, these three were patients I actually thought I was treating adequately.—*Todd Lininger, M.D.*

I took an alternate road in medicine because of multiple disasters I witnessed in medical school, like patients being killed unintentionally. Everywhere I turned it was iatrogenic mayhem. So I decided that I would pursue a path of medicine that honored

and holding grudges. Their experience of frustration and impatience with situations or co-workers might pass without being mentioned, but the internalized energetic dynamic can reappear as muscle tension, headaches, insomnia, or digestive disturbances.

About ten years ago I had an office manager named **Samuel Morris**. He took over the job following a rapid turnover of employees who had proved to be unsuited for the position, and had left the office in a chaotic state. Samuel jumped into his work and, with little supervision and in a remarkably short time, created a new organization for the projects involved in our teaching activities. He developed a very tidy computer filing system and formalized protocols for activities we repeated every teaching season. Samuel is a doodler and a tapper. Any spare scraps of paper on his desk were covered with artistic doodles that he executed while talking on the telephone. When not doodling he tapped his pen against the desktop, twitched his feet, and crossed and uncrossed his legs. He had worn glasses for reading since early childhood. Samuel also got very bad headaches, sometimes preventing him from doing any work, headaches clearly triggered by muscle spasms in his mid-back and neck. When working under pressure for a long period he became impatient and even rude with me and with the students on the telephone. His muscles grew tighter and his headaches intensified.

From time to time, Samuel asked me to treat him. These treatments always helped, but Samuel's biopsychotype persistently catapulted him back into active symptoms whenever we were working against a deadline. He instinctively resolved much of his problem with two lifestyle decisions: he cut back to part-time work, and he got a dog. Bringing the dog to work required that Samuel walk him several times during the day, and he also took the time to take the dog for a run in the park at the end of his work day.

the Hippocratic oath and at least didn't hurt anybody. Acupuncture satisfies my need for a method that works metaphysically as well as physically.—*John Adams, M.D.*
My inaugural experience as an acupuncturist was with my daughter. She was born at twenty-six weeks and required surgery to close an open duct in her heart. She couldn't be weaned off the respirator after surgery because half of her diaphragm was paralyzed. Presented with a list of horrible options, we decided to bring an acupunc-

Grudges and Explosions

A person with additional Fire in his constitution can move quickly from frustration to irritability to an inability to hold his temper in check. This sort of person has difficulty keeping criticism of co-workers and superiors to himself. He will have an uncanny ability to recall, without apparent thought or effort, any and all past insults and injuries, as if they had been catalogued in an emotional database. He may explode in anger when he reaches a stress overload or perceives one too many insults to his excitable psyche. Such a person can be productive in an office or team situation, but can be unpredictable and sometimes unpleasant. In extreme cases, the irritability and resentment escalate and become intolerable in the workplace, or ordinary family and social situations. The evolution from frustration and irritability to explosive anger is described as stagnant Liver Qi creating "rising Liver Fire." Fire's nature is to rise, hence the escalation from simmering resentment to unrestrained anger.

Erik Stendahl, an emergency physician from the midwest, was a student in my medical acupuncture training program. Part of the training experience is for each physician to be a patient — to be interviewed, evaluated, examined, discussed, and treated by a group of physician colleagues in the class. Erik lives on a hundred-acre farm that is completely surrounded with a border of trees. The driveway to his house is a half-mile long. He takes pride in his abilities as an emergency physician and as the founding administrator of his emergency room. He also holds a certain pride in the distance he keeps from other people, and says that he is happiest when he's at home riding his horse. The problems he presented during his interview included insomnia, teeth-grinding at night, and intermittent but vague problems with digestion, such as bloating one day and diarrhea the next. He also acknowledged that he commonly grows impatient working with nurses or other

---

turist into the intensive care nursery. He worked out a treatment plan to be done by tapping at points on her back with a tiny hammer that had needles in it. He wanted this to be done between 3:00 and 5:00 in the morning, which is the time of maximum energetic activity of the lungs. Every other night I trotted into the intensive care nursery and tap-tap-tapped at the points. After doing this for a week we started to see return of function. In another week she was off the ventilator and went home after

doctors and prefers to rely on his own competence and independence. And he clearly remembers the insults and offenses that he perceives from others in his life, at work and at home.

On physical examination, the muscles across the front of Erik's chest, his shoulders, and front and sides of his neck were firm and tightly contracted. They were painful to our probing fingers, and the tightness limited how far he could turn his head or bend his neck. We discussed his history, the physical findings, and his work and social situation as a group, listening to each student's observations and proposed diagnosis and treatments. After thirty minutes of this discussion our patient stood up, eyes bulging and face flushed, and shouted with clear frustration and anger: *"Will you please finish your goddamn talking so we can get on with the goddamn treatment!"* We promptly concluded our analysis and treated him with a needle pattern to calm rising Liver Fire.

Anxiety and Emotional Paralysis

Just as stagnant Liver Qi can boil into anger, it can also simmer internally as intensifying anxiety. This anxiety occurs in people with constitutions similar to the emergency physician above, but who lack the innate confidence of their more outgoing counterparts. Their anxiety grows internally as timidity inhibiting their self-expression, and can eventually evolve into a state of emotional paralysis. (Renee Carter fits more into this profile than any of the others above.) Anxiety drives them to use guises to avoid being noticed and especially to avoid making eye contact: blending invisibly into groups, covering their eyes with tinted or dark glasses (often claiming to suffer from "sensitive eyes"), wearing their hair long over their eyes, or using hand gestures to cover the mouth or face while talking. They commonly suffer ongoing physical symptoms of

she gained weight. She has turned out okay.—*Brian Bouch, M.D.*
In stark contrast to much of what I was force fed and had to memorize in medical school, acupuncture is a system that makes sense to me intuitively. I could explain most of it easily to a ten-year-old.—*Howard Silverman, M.D.*
For me, acupuncture has been a breath of fresh air and a whole new system of medicine, a real symbol of hope for the future of healing.—*Martha Grout, M.D.*

stagnant and obstructed blood that result from the stagnant psychological Qi. These symptoms can include chronically tight and woody muscles, headaches, or unpredictable menstrual or digestive disturbances.

Esther Jacobson, who retired early from her nursing supervisor position when her attorney husband retired from his practice, came to see me with a thirty-year history of crippling migraine headaches. The headaches started when she was raising her young family as a divorced working mother. At the time she saw me, she was having headaches as often as four to six times a month, each one putting her to bed for one to three days. They were triggered by direct sunlight, flashing bright lights, inadequate sleep, chocolate, and coffee. She had been evaluated by headache specialists five times, but their medications did not break the recurring cycle.

Esther did not consider herself an anxious or tightly-wired person. She held a lot of tension in her neck and shoulder muscles, and described the headache pattern as originating in the muscle just over her right shoulder blade, then rising to the back of her neck and through her head to her right eye. Esther had spent her life trying to keep everything moving: her family, her hospital staff, her second husband's demanding schedule, and her crippling headaches. She did not express her frustration, irritability, or anxiety, but she certainly experienced these emotions during the different stages of her life. Rather than reacting to her difficult circumstances with explosions of impatience or anger, she forced those emotions inside, only for them to emerge as recurring headaches.

People in the workplace with prominent Vision/Action constitutional features usually sense when they are anxious or irritable, and, for professional interactions, keep these tendencies in check. Depending upon the intensity of their anxiety and their state of fatigue, they might not be as diligent reining in these dynamics in their personal lives. Others

My patients accepted acupuncture eagerly and my practice grew quickly because the acupuncture was doing what it is supposed to do.—*Lowell Kobrin, M.D., Ph.D.*
I was certainly one of the most traditional physicians in the clinical section of the acupuncture program. I think half the other physicians in the room were into some type of complementary practice, and were merely adding acupuncture to their armamentarium. I remember the gasp I heard when we were introducing ourselves on the

who have not been required to develop a professional or social persona might fail to recognize the role that anxiety plays in their internal and social dynamics. They might simply consider it as innate timidity or reluctance to draw attention to themselves, or, at the opposite extreme, as impulsiveness or bad temper.

To repeat, the four disturbance patterns that I see most often in the Vision/Action types are fidgeting, impatience and tight muscles, grudges and explosions, and emotional paralysis. As I teach this biopsychotype to physicians, I always see nodding heads and smiles of recognition as doctors identify themselves or their spouses in this terrain, or as the description explains the behavior of colleagues and patients. Most of us can see some part of ourselves in these descriptions, some of us will recognize a good deal of ourselves in one of them. Certainly we can all recognize people we know in some of the more exaggerated forms.

Potential Behavior in the Vision/Action Biopsychotype

With all three acupuncture biopsychotypes there are no absolute and fixed patterns of manifestation. There are no rules that require a standard combination of characteristics and disturbances to qualify for a Vision/Action constitution. Each individual possesses unique qualities and characteristics, and an equally unique collection of disturbances and symptoms. Understanding our own constitutions and disturbances enlightens us about our family's health heritage and about how our health may evolve through time.

Each of the four common Vision/Action patterns above, or any combination of these patterns, can occur intermittently and transiently in an otherwise healthy and integrated person. They can also be the norm of a person's character. Or, with time, stress, illness, and fatigue

---

first day and I mentioned that I implanted spinal cord stimulators. You would have thought that I was the quack in the group! I also realized that many of the people in that room were more interested in caring for their patients than in making more money. It was very refreshing.—*Todd Lininger, M.D.*
My job is writing and editing science articles. Every time I come to your office I feel that I am setting medical science back another fifty years. Needles! Cupping! Scrap-

they can evolve in intensity, duration, or complexity of symptoms, both psychoemotional and physical. One of the remarkable features of this constitution is the variability, and sometimes vagueness, of symptom combinations. This phenomenon is especially challenging when most of a person's symptoms are showing in their early stages, without an organ being clearly disordered. Such people risk being labeled as hypochondriacal by friends and physicians, whereas they are probably showing disturbances in some of the quiet functions of the autonomic nervous system at the same time as suffering from muscle contractions and other problems of obstructed Qi.

Stress and Tension Exaggerations

"Ambitious" and "competitive" are terms sometimes used to describe the decisive and driven qualities seen in this biopsychotype. In sports, Vision/Action competitiveness shows up in the passion for movement and challenge rather than as an indomitable drive to win. The Vision/Action terrain is usually the first to express symptoms triggered by the stress and tension in our lives. These patterns occur commonly in many people dealing with the demands of modern life. The anxiety and anger that accompany chronic Liver Qi stagnation may manifest simply as a moody, critical, and irritable personality or, in more pronounced states, as a foul-tempered or bloody-minded character. If the frustration is severe, the consequences can be dangerous.

The most extreme disturbance in the Vision/Action constitution occurs when internal tension, accumulated from longstanding stagnant Liver Qi, explodes in a violent or brutal expression. This rising Liver Fire is characterized by extreme and uncontrollable anxiety and frustration. It can start as distension in the abdomen, fullness or pain below the

---

ing! But it works. I feel so much better. I have more energy. I can walk straighter and sleep better. But I don't mention it to my colleagues.—*Paul Bendix*
I can't understand why there were so many nonbelievers when the proof was so evident in the healing. People looked askance when I told them of my success or my wife's success with acupuncture. However, skepticism has diminished appreciably in the last five years. Acupuncture has become white bread.—*Bill Kane*

ribcage, or a lump in the throat. The Fire moves rapidly to create red eyes or a red face and culminates in a crippling headache or explosive and unrestrained anger. (Think of the expression "blowing your top.") Rising Liver Fire can also be the culprit behind impulsive, offensive driving, and road rage.

Liver is responsible for planning. If the Liver vitality is depleted, symptoms such as lack of direction, inability to plan, and indecisiveness can emerge. Liver-depleted people can express anxiety by finding problems with every situation, continually analyzing but without resolving the problems or moving forward. These symptoms represent the opposite end of the Vision/Action spectrum, where Liver function is depleted rather than agitated.

Liver energy is responsible for the eyes and vision, fingernails and toenails. Therefore, problems with vision commonly afflict people of this constitution. Vision/Action types may need reading glasses as early as primary school, or for distance vision at the time of puberty. Other symptoms can include dry eyes, floaters, and blurred vision when fatigued. In later life, cataracts, retinal detachment, and macular degeneration can develop. The vitality of the Liver is reflected in the strength of the fingernails and toenails. People with disturbed Liver function commonly complain of soft nails that bend or break easily, ridged nails, and cuticles that become inflamed easily. Patients can develop soft nails following prolonged courses of medications such as antibiotics or corticosteroids. The nails might never return to their pre-treatment condition. From the perspective of acupuncture pathology, the medications have altered the vitality of the Liver, and this weakness is reflected in the nails.

To someone who is just beginning acupuncture: do not expect a quick fix. An illness that took years for you to feel will not be fixed in one treatment. I believe that the patterns of illness are embedded in the body and memory. Thus, if you have a chronic condition as I did, you may need to recondition not only your body but also your mind, so that the mind can create new patterns of health to replace the old ones. The improvement in the body will follow after that.—*Katrina Radke*

Muscles, tendons, and ligaments, the tissues that allow us to move and be active, are the most common targets of stress and tension. The sides of the head, trunk, and legs – the lateral surfaces of the body – are the body zones most influenced by the Vision/Action channels. Liver-Gall Bladder energy allows for the physical movement so characteristic of this biopsychotype, as well as the agility and confidence often perceived by others as physical recklessness.

I knew **Alan Davidov** in medical school. He was focused and ambitious as he defined and executed each step that led him to specialize in reconstructive surgery. He was an accomplished athlete and received a partial scholarship to play lacrosse while in medical school. He had worn glasses since puberty. Alan was sufficiently aware of his internal tension to learn transcendental meditation to help him relax during medical training.

Alan appeared in my office thirty years after our graduation. His wife, a professional dancer familiar with the value of acupuncture for the muscular problems encountered in her discipline, forced him to make the appointment. He related his story in crisp medical terms: recurrent low back pain, now chronic and prohibiting him from playing competitive racquetball, and burning pain radiating into his buttocks and thigh while sitting in administration meetings at his medical group, helped temporarily with anti-inflammatory drugs and sedatives to relax the muscles.

He had already dismissed physical therapy and acupuncture as being of no value after two sessions of each, and, impatient to make the pain go away, underwent a surgical decompression of a vertebral disk. The surgery did not help the symptoms; nor, fortunately, did it make them worse.

"Does the stress of your surgical or administrative duties affect the pain?"

The first day, the first week, I felt shaken up internally, but in a good way. I didn't feel destabilized, but jostled, and I liked that. It felt like it was the right thing to do. I felt a little bit exhilarated, a little bit tired, and very encouraged. The treatments created a state of clear-headedness, the kind of moments I get when I'm writing well. There is a translucency, a transparency, and I feel wonderful, entranced. I recognize my limits and boundaries, but do not feel my expectations and possibilities restricted by them.

"Yes, of course. Especially when I'm frustrated dealing with the stuffy bastards I have to work with in administration. But I'd never let them know that they aggravated the pain in my butt."

As he relaxed into our new relationship, Alan revealed more features that fit perfectly with the Vision/Action biopsychotype: glasses since puberty; dry eyes as an adult; chronic fungus under four toenails; always active in competitive sports and frustrated when he wasn't able to be physically active; rapidly insightful in organizational planning and impatient with colleagues who didn't agree with him; prone to foot tapping, sweaty palms, and pacing; pounding heart when under pressure; several recent bouts of atrial fibrillation (a deregulation of the heart's rhythmic beating, under control of the ANS) when especially anxious; and everything made worse with more than one cup of coffee a day.

He noticed improvement after his first treatment, even though he had been very skeptical of acupuncture's value for his condition. I asked him to keep a pain diary so we could track the circumstances when the pain disappeared or intensified. Keeping the diary for two months confirmed that the greatest triggers were the administrative meetings and confrontations with colleagues who did not see solutions as quickly as he did. He started having long pain-free periods after three treatments and gradually returned to more physical activity. He began playing racquetball again, pain-free. He now understands how his sitting posture and his psychological tension affect the back pain and recognizes that acupuncture can help relieve and prevent emotional and muscle stress and irritation. He returns periodically for treatment whenever he anticipates an especially stressful event or when he needs to recover from one.

And that is very different from how I felt when my trigeminal neuralgia was being treated with drugs.—*Joe DiPrisco*

Learning medical acupuncture taught me to see and hear patients. It has reshaped the way I think about patient diagnosis and treatment. It has not negated anything I learned in medical school; rather, it greatly expanded my medical consciousness. Before I took medical acupuncture training, I saw the patient from the bottom of the

In addition to injuries that occur while in motion, the muscular problems seen most frequently in this biopsychotype come from inflammation and spasm. These conditions result from sluggish Qi not moving blood through the tissues, leaving them stagnant and irritated. This state creates muscle tension patterns that can originate in the middle of the back and climb to the shoulders and neck and just stay there, leaving them stiff and achy. The pattern can degenerate into a muscle tension headache that starts in the back of the neck and marches over the scalp to the eye. The tension can dig into the sides of the neck, tightening the muscles of the jaw, causing jaw clenching during the day and teeth grinding at night. The irritation can also start in the middle of the belly and climb to the chest and create symptoms similar to an ulcer or a heart attack. Or it can move from the chest to the front of the neck. Or anywhere else there are muscles. Once a myofascial (muscle and connective tissue) spasm and inflammation pattern is set up, it loves to return to the same place and intensify when we reach a state of stress or fatigue, especially if we have not been stretching or exercising regularly. And it can stay around for such a long time that the texture of the muscle tissue changes from soft and flexible to hard and knotty. Like Wood. Does this remind you of yourself or anyone you know?

The Liver stores and releases blood during times of rest and activity, and therefore plays a role in menstruation. Liver and Vision/Action disturbance should be considered as a contributing culprit in women with premenstrual pain, scant or heavy bleeding, irregular periods, fertility problems, or endometriosis. All such problems can be addressed, at least initially, by restoring balance to the Vision/Action circuit.

---

mountain. After I took it, I saw the patient from the top of the mountain. Acupuncture allowed me to see that we cannot just lump people into big statistical groups. We must take into consideration the constitution and lifestyle of the patient as well.— *Lowell Kobrin, M.D., Ph.D.*

When my regular doctor said he couldn't do anything more for my pain, he suggested I see you. I knew you were an M.D. who practiced acupuncture, but I was intimidated.

Other general features of the Vision/Action type are linked to agitation of the autonomic nervous system and its interaction with Liver Qi. Typical symptoms include nervous sweating, moist palms, a jumpy restlessness, and nervous habits such as nail and cuticle chewing, fiddling with hair, twisting fingers, wringing hands, and sighing, in addition to the incessant finger tapping, pen clicking, and foot bouncing. Dizziness, insomnia, frequent tension headaches, easy sensitivity to foods and medications and changes in the weather, and a sensation of pounding or racing in the heart are also potential symptoms. And, finally, stress can generate an imprecise migrating abdominal discomfort, along with other digestive symptoms such as sensitive appetite, belching, regurgitation of food, nausea, or relentless churning in the abdomen. The abdominal symptoms are often diagnosed as aspects of "irritable bowel syndrome."

Wood and Fire, Alcohol and Coffee

The elements of Wood and Fire are affiliated with Liver - Gall Bladder and Master of the Heart - Triple Heater. The color affinity acknowledged by those of predominantly Liver or Wood makeup is blue or blue-green, a turquoise color rather than midnight blue. Their flavor affinity is for sour or citrus, such as grapefruit, vinegar, or an acid taste. Their preferred season is spring, the season in which symptoms noticeably improve or worsen. Sensitivity to the wind can also be a feature in this constitution: feeling either exhilarated and invigorated or exhausted and fatigued after a walk on a windy day reflects both extremes of this sensitivity.

I couldn't think of anything but voodoo. I was scared to death of all those needles. But at the first visit I was very impressed that you were unpretentious and said to try it a few times and then evaluate what acupuncture might be able to do. You said, I can't cure you, but I think I can improve the quality of your life.—*Johnny Maddox*
Many people I know are scared to come for acupuncture. My husband couldn't do it. The very idea of needles! They don't understand that it is a very gentle procedure.

Vision/Action people with a predominance of Fire tend to prefer the color red, bitter or burned flavors (such as heavily-roasted peppers, very dark toast, and well-grilled vegetables), and summer, and they will either love or hate a hot climate. The Fire affinities are less commonly encountered in the Vision/Action constitution than are those of Wood.

Alcohol is the mood changer of choice in many people with this anxiety and anger quality, because alcohol temporarily calms the Liver, relaxes emotional irritability, and moves Qi and blood. The impact of alcohol on Liver energy and tissue, however, is not salutary when used regularly to excess, for it creates a chronic inflammatory condition that accentuates the irritability caused originally by stagnant Liver Qi. Interestingly, patients who have taken a prolonged course of a medication that is potentially toxic to the liver, such as some antifungal, antiviral, or anti-inflammatory agents, report being aware of an increase in irritability or anxiety. This can occur while they are using the medication or after they've stopped, even if the liver function blood tests have remained normal.

Vision/Action types commonly flirt dangerously with caffeinated products: coffee, black or green tea, cola and other caffeine-fortified carbonated drinks, and dark chocolate. Their physiologic and energetic nature attracts them to these stimulants. Most will insist that a cup or two of coffee is indispensable in the morning, just to get going. Others will have an additional cup if they wake up with a headache, knowing that the extra jolt of caffeine has a good shot at easing the headache. And many will candidly say that they crave the buzz, the charge, the focus of attention that comes from the caffeine. It helps them get their projects done. But they also know that the extra caffeine adds to their muscle

---

There is a profundity that comes with the acupuncture treatment; like a meditation, a serenity, a kind of spiritual event.—*Joan Kip*

I was skeptical regarding acupuncture. California has seen so many medical fads over the years, and I expected little from my treatments. But I had instant results from my first treatment. I found immediate relief from the pain in my back that my unbalanced walk always triggered. And a welcome absence of side effects. The absence of

tension, their jaw clenching, their headaches, impatience, insomnia, and blood pressure problems. Yet, changing their caffeine habit is a challenge most are reluctant to take on.

You have probably recognized some of yourself in this tour of the various expressions of the Vision/Action biopsychotype. If you're impatient to find out how strongly these qualities play in your constitution, take a look at Chapter 8. You'll gain a good appreciation of just how much Vision/Action you have in your makeup. But don't jump to any conclusions yet. Continue reading the next two chapters – on Nurture/Duty and Will/Spirit. You'll certainly find some of yourself there as well.

---

grogginess from pain medications was wonderful, because for someone like me whose stamina is already severely taxed by hemiplegia, even the effects of aspirin can be unwelcome.—*Paul Bendix*
I can remember saying to you in an early interview when you asked about my emotional state, that I can get depressed, not a depressive personality, but that I can get depressed. I am fascinated by this approach that can group these families of symp-

toms just through talking and observation. Most of the doctors I have seen are strict scientists, not artists or healers.—*Mary Wilson*
The needles don't seem to hurt at all. Obviously I feel them, but mostly I feel the pressure of your fingers on my skin, then a faint sting. As you manipulate the needle I feel a sense of fullness in that area. I wouldn't call it an ache, rather a fullness. After the first few needles I feel my body starting to relax, and I go into this kind of altered state.—*Julie Mendosa*

CHAPTER 6

NURTURE/DUTY BIOPSYCHOTYPE

Renee Carter was the ideal patient to introduce you to some of the fundamental ideas of acupuncture, and especially the frustration–tension–muscle dynamic so prominent in the Vision/Action biopsychotype. To explore the attributes of the Nurture/Duty type, let's bring back Bill Kane and Mary Wilson, whom you met in Chapter 4. Bill and Mary overlap in some of their Nurture/Duty features. But when it comes to exaggerations of behavior and manifestations of imbalance, they move in different directions. Their differences have to do with the qualities of Earth and Metal.

Bill Kane described himself at our first interview many years ago as *"an Irish-Catholic alcoholic Democrat, Wagner-loving, bridge playing beach bum, someone who has always enjoyed his life (and you may print that, Dr. Helms)."* He consistently embodies the features of the exuberant Nurture/Duty person: lively, inclusive of the people around them, and fun to be with. His love of opera is infectious to everyone who knows him. He started an opera club for his friends and solicited contributions from alcohol and cigarette companies (with whom he had professional ties) so the members could have the best seats in the house.

Mary Wilson is also of the Nurture/Duty fabric, but a different pattern than Bill. Her initial complaint was thirty years of recurrent bronchitis with regular thick sputum, combined with a chronically draining ear infection. Additionally, she has had mild acne on her face and over much of her chest and back since puberty. Mary's style at our initial meeting was straightforward, no-nonsense reporting that quickly shifted into self-deprecating humor. We laughed about the genetic catastrophe underlying her condition and that no one else in her family had been born with such frail health. She called it *"piss poor protoplasm, poorly put together."* She spends no time feeling sorry for

---

I like the moxa. It heats up the needles, it warms the area, and it is soothing and calming. The heat penetrates through the needles, depending on the vigor of the person delivering the moxa. My mother used to adore the moxa. I sometimes thought that was the only reason she was coming. For me, it's the icing on the cake.—*Elena Verde*
It's great. Somehow I can feel the connection between the needles and the channels and the inside of my body. I feel that blockages are being opened and something is

herself and has always been active in church and community activities, feeling that she wants *"to give back and help others."* Even in her retirement, she continues to sing in the church choir and help with the education programs at her neighborhood community center.

Earth and Metal

A common thread of Nurture and Duty runs through both Bill and Mary: giving and caring, whether through the opera club or community activities. The differences between these two derive from their main elements: Bill embodies Earth; Mary embodies Metal.

Earth gives us the food that provides all nourishment. It symbolizes fertility and fullness of provisions. Earth offers a foundation on which to build and grow, the ground that supports us all. Earth is the source of the four other elements and, as such, represents the center of balance among the elements. The time of year associated with Earth is harvest, or Indian summer, a season of transition and transformation, the center of the year.

Bill Kane exemplifies the nurturing qualities of a predominantly Earth personality. He radiates the aura of a man who enjoys sensual pleasures to an extreme – music, food, drink, and social gatherings. His magnetic personality and generosity of spirit draw those who meet him into his very pleasant universe.

Metal represents structural strength, support, and reinforcement. Not always warm or life-giving like the other elements, Metal is nevertheless important because of its durability and its function of creating structure from matter. It can follow the form of a mold. It can be rigid, or flexible, or hard and brittle. Duty and responsibility are foremost qualities in a Metal person. The season associated with Metal is autumn, the time of maturity and change.

---

being released. A pathway to my soul is opened, and that appeals to me. I always feel exhilarated, and very hopeful.—*Joe DiPrisco*

Acupuncture is an awkward and invasive experience. But it is also tremendously relaxing, restoring, and refreshing. It is a strange fugue state to be lying for ten minutes with needles in, with the quadrants pulsing away. It's like a yoga pose that puts you in direct contact with your body, a connection that you have to otherwise make an effort

Mary Wilson clearly displays Metallic qualities in the strength of her character as well as in her physical problems. Although herself handicapped, she taught handicapped children for decades, and, although hearing-impaired from the chronic ear infection, she sings in the choir and takes her grandchildren to the symphony. She has problems with her lungs, which are Metal organs.

Creation and Movement of Qi

The Spleen, Lungs, Stomach, and Large Intestine are the organs associated with the Nurture/Duty biopsychotype. From an acupuncture perspective, these are also the crucial organs in the creation and movement of Qi. This constitutional terrain is concerned with the fundamental nurturing and day-to-day survival of the organism. Stomach and Large Intestine – the digestive system – are the hollow organs through which the process of digestion takes place. Spleen's role is to extract and direct energy generated through the digestion. Lung's role is to refine and move that energy by means of respiration. Qi is the driving force in all physiological processes. When Qi is ample and flowing we have good health. When Qi is weak or stagnant we experience disorder and disturbance in health.

The Spleen-digestive territory of this biopsychotype is associated with the element Earth. The Lung-respiratory territory is associated with the element Metal. People composed primarily of the Nurture/ Duty biopsychotype typically manifest many overlaps of Earth and Metal qualities, with one of them predominating. But the characteristics of the two poles are distinct enough to warrant understanding both of these labels. Simply put, Earth represents stability, being grounded, and creating a nourishing environment. A person of predominantly Earth composition is balanced, centered, and sympathetic, and works harmo-

---

to get to. It feels like having had a big night's sleep and being really relaxed without any creaks and tensions anywhere. Just stimulating the energy to move around in the body is useful. The energy knows what to do. The body knows how to heal itself or take what it needs, to a certain point.—*Mary Ellen Hannibal*
When you do the treatment with electricity I notice how I can relax more, especially with the buzzes [high-frequency stimulation]. I've never had a problem with the buzz.

niously with his environment. Metal signifies durability, infrastructure, and order. A person of predominantly Metal composition is organized, disciplined, meticulous, reliable, and precise.

Nurture/Duty people are typically calm, clean, and neat in appearance and fastidious regarding their personal surroundings. They like order and reliably fulfill their obligations. Those with a predominance of Earth qualities are usually round and fleshy in build, have soothing and melodic voices, and are sensitive to flavors and odors. They have a psychological predisposition to nurturing and caring for the people in their lives, both personal and professional. Men and women of predominantly Earth makeup elevate parenting and the nuclear family above all other commitments and values. There is also an exuberant expression of the Earth type as a bon vivant, knowledgeable about food and wine, who knows how to enjoy and share life's sensual pleasures. He emanates a fullness of presence and spirit that can be quite magnetic.

Those with a predominance of Metal qualities tend to have a thinner build, often with angular features. They display an authoritative, matter-of-fact affect rather than the melodic voice of their Earth counterparts. They are extremely conscientious about fulfilling their real or perceived responsibilities. Dedicated to participating in good works, they have a strong sense of duty and are often active in civic or religious pursuits. People dominated by Metal qualities can be perceived as unemotional, usually because they are so absorbed in the responsibilities of life and duties of work.

Functions and Influences of the Spleen and Stomach

Acupuncture classical literature describes healthy Spleen Qi as something we can feel throughout our bodies, the energy that provides

---

The beeps [low frequency stimulation] build up the strength, but can be unpleasant if I'm feeling sensitive. So the combination of the needles and the beeps and buzzes and moxa is the whole treatment of acupuncture. And when I'm hurting and tired I know I need all of it.—*Mary Johnson*

I feel a shift in the relationship as I begin an acupuncture treatment. I am more deeply connected with my patient and we are truly working as a team. It's as if I am engaged

the mental and physical vitality to take on and complete projects at work and in life. Spleen's sphere of influence includes our capacity for concentrating, focusing, and memorizing. Spleen also influences the lips and mouth, the vitality of muscles, the sense of touch, and it is responsible for keeping blood inside the vessels. Spleen and Earth are associated with yellow and earth tones, and sweet flavors. Spleen and Stomach are viewed as one inseparable unit in acupuncture physiology. In fact, the Spleen supervises the entire digestive tract and all digestive processes from mouth to rectum.

In acupuncture physiology, the Spleen's most important function is directing digestion, primarily in the Stomach, by transporting the nutritional essence from foods and liquids from the Stomach to the Lung. This seems an unusual concept when viewed from our western understanding of the physiology of digestion; however, it is a critical step in the acupuncture understanding of creating and moving Qi in the body. When food and drink arrive in the Stomach, acids and enzymes break them down. The fermentation process prepares the nourishment for the Spleen, which separates the usable part from the unusable. The Stomach sends the unusable part downward into the intestines, where it undergoes further fermentation, separation, and utilization or excretion.

The Spleen extracts the pure, energetic essence from nourishment and thereby generates most of the Qi that flows to the other organs and tissues of the body. This Spleen Qi, in the traditional Chinese concept of energy physiology, moves to the Lung, where it combines with the pure energy from inhaled air. The combination of Spleen Qi and Lung Qi makes up the "nourishing energy" that is propelled by the rhythmic respirations of the Lung to the skin, muscles, and organs.

---

in performing energetic surgery on them. There is an easy intimacy that develops, and patients relish the sense of well being and relaxation that accompanies the treatments.—*Howard Silverman, M.D.*
Acupuncture for me became a spiritual adventure. When you become whole, then it is a spiritual enterprise. I can depend on the acupuncture to help with the coming together. I feel myself flowing, despite age impediments, keeping open. I sense it.

The Spleen fulfills other functions in traditional acupuncture physiology, the most important of which are keeping blood inside the arteries, veins, and capillaries; nourishing the muscles; and holding the internal organs in their proper places. If the Spleen and Lung function well, there will be good appetite, good digestion, regular bowel movements, healthy organs, easy menstrual periods, strong muscles, good concentration and memory, and plenty of vitality for all of life's responsibilities.

If your constitution is predominantly the balanced Spleen-Stomach-Earth form of the Nurture/Duty biopsychotype, you likely have a rosy complexion, moist lips, and a welcoming smile. You are full-bodied, easygoing, generous, kind, compassionate, and tolerant. You like to eat and probably enjoy preparing food and serving others. You like to touch and be touched and enjoy a hug when greeting your friends. Your caring nature makes you find time to listen to and help solve the challenges your friends face in their personal lives and the challenges your colleagues face at work. You have a good memory for the details in the lives of your family, friends, and colleagues, and you exercise good practical sense as you find solutions to problems.

You love sweet flavors in fruits, carbohydrates, and especially milk chocolate. Because of your attraction to sweets, you constantly struggle to maintain a reasonable weight. You might express your caring and compassion in one-on-one circumstances. Or you might swell with the spirit of the moment and invite everyone near you to participate in your enjoyment, whether it is a good meal, a new wine, another round at the bar, or any other form of pleasure-enhancement. You endorse the motto: More is better.

It flows. I just sense it. It is like a meditation. I believe if the body is rested and not stopped up, there is much more energy to be creative.—*Joan Kip*
There is something sacred about putting needles in someone and how you treat them after the needles are in. After I contact the Qi I always put a calming hand on the patient so they know that I know what they felt, and I get it. That's very calming for them.—*Kirk Pappas, M.D.*

Bill Kane has enjoyed life to the most unbridled exaggerations of this constitution. An alcoholic for many years, by retirement age his liver was turning cirrhotic, and his lungs were emphysematous from a lifetime of smoking. He takes good care of his exterior body with some bodybuilding and exercise, and verges on exhibitionism when he gets to the beach. He has a refined taste in food, people, drink, and travel, and wants all those he touches to feast with him in his pleasures.

Functions and Influences of the Lung

The most important consequence of respiration is to impel Qi through the acupuncture channels to all the tissues of the body. The Lung takes in air and extracts pure Qi, combines it with the Spleen Qi, and in turn propels it as nourishing energy throughout the body. The Lung helps to maintain the body's warmth and vitality through this circulation of Qi. The protective energy in the surface channels flows through the skin and outermost layer of muscles. Protective energy creates an energetic barrier that defends the muscles and organs against damage by extremes or changes in climate. Without this protection, weather extremes of heat or cold, damp or dry, or even wind, can have a damaging effect on an organ that is susceptible to these external conditions.

Chinese classics describe the skin as a third lung, and the quality of the skin mirrors the vitality of Lung energy. The Lung spreads Qi and fluid through the body, thereby ensuring a healthy glow to the skin and a healthy quality to the body hair. The Lung's sphere of influence also encompasses the nose and throat and vocal cords, the sense of smell, and the strength of the voice. People of Lung-Metal composition will

---

The treatment itself can actually be pleasant, which is delightful for patients and liberating for doctors. I extinguish the glaring overhead light, turn on a low side light, and apply the needles. I manipulate the needles, attend to my patient's comfort, and gradually withdraw myself, allowing the patient to enter his acupuncture space. Frequently they fall asleep. One patient told me that during her treatment she dreamed she was in a Swiss village with an inch of snow over everything, shining in the moon-

commonly enjoy autumn, have an affinity for white, and prefer flavorful seasoning. Likewise, such people may find that autumn is the season when respiratory problems are most likely to emerge.

If your constitution is the balanced Lung-Metal form of the Nurture/Duty biopsychotype, you are likely to be slimmer of build than your round Spleen-Earth Nurture/Duty counterpart described above, and your hands and fingers are long and slender, not fleshy. Your complexion may be paler and your appetites more restrained, yet you share your counterpart's orderliness and sense of responsibility. You are organized, rational, thrifty, and observant. Your strengths include unwavering loyalty and a strong sense of duty. You possess, privately or professionally, a dedication to a pursuit or organization that you elevate above your own individual needs and interests. You seek quality and perfection, use words to exactly express your ideas, and have a good memory. You have a keen but restrained sense of humor and give the impression of likeable equilibrium.

Disciplined and organized in your undertakings, you are most likely a creature of habit and routine. You are respectful of established order. Because you appear calm and reflective and rarely upset, those around you might consider you to be detached or unemotional. You generally react with reason when confronting conflict, analyzing the problems facing you with an intellectual abstraction. You are probably aware of a tendency to a melancholy mood, but you refuse to allow this to interfere with executing your responsibilities. Most likely you have very tidy, small handwriting. When your digestive system is in good order you like your food to be interesting and flavorful, maybe tending toward spicy and hot.

---

light. I consider that a job well done.—*Richard Zweig, M.D.*
My fifteen-year practice of karate taught me that much of the success of karate performance, of the body's inherent abilities, depends on the movement and utilization of the energy force called Qi. Qi was a great mystery to me, and I became obsessed with a desire to learn more about how to strengthen it, control it, direct it. Therefore it seemed reasonable to enroll in an acupuncture class that taught about Qi. Until this point I had

While **Mary Wilson's** biopsychotype is clearly the Lung-Metal division of Nurture/Duty, the innate physical strength of her lungs has never been strong. Her discipline and dedication to doing good works demonstrate the psychological strength of her Lung energy, as she expresses the Duty inherent in this type. Her physical problems, on the contrary, manifest in the territories that Lung governs: skin, lungs, and sinuses; susceptibility to respiratory infections; and the absence of a robust vitality.

Exaggerations in the Mental and Emotional Levels of Nurture/Duty

Qualities of the diverse subdivisions of the Nurture/Duty biopsychotype overlap in the same person more commonly than do the subdivisions of the other two biopsychotypes. While it is common to find strengths and weaknesses of both poles in one person, it is likely that either the Spleen-Earth features or the Lung-Metal features will define the bulk of one's personality and biological traits. If, as you work through the questions in Chapter 8 or the questionnaire in Appendix II, you find many of the Nurture/Duty qualities in yourself, don't be surprised if they include aspects of both the Spleen and Lung territories of influence. That's the way the body works. Few people are purely one or the other.

Exaggerations of the healthy qualities of this biopsychotype commonly occur in the personality and behavior of Nurture/Duty types. The psychological exaggerations can evolve into serious problems. If they are prolonged, or especially if they are intensified through physical illness, they can develop into more difficult emotional problems or enduring physical symptoms.

---

never considered using acupuncture in my gynecology practice.—*Robert Chase, M.D.*
My friends say I look wonderful, and I tell them that acupuncture is the most important thing that helped me. I wouldn't be walking as well if I didn't have acupuncture. It opens up my entire body. There's a great sense of relaxation after every session, and I feel like I'm flowing smoothly again. I feel much more whole starting the next day, and that maintains itself for at least a month. If I can go once a month, my arthri-

Take, for example, the nurturing quality of the Earth Mother type. When her focus is on raising her family and caring for her home, caring and supporting are the healthiest possible expressions of Nurture/Duty qualities. If, however, these care-giving qualities are offered to members of the extended family, the neighbors, the church, and people at the office, the nurturing type can easily lose herself in solving everyone's problems and trying to keep everyone happy. At some point along this trajectory of generosity, the caregiver starts to deplete herself. Yet she might – because of these very qualities – feel obligated or responsible to follow through with every complicated and needy situation (or worry about their welfare if she can't help them), even at the cost to her own emotional and physical well-being. It is this state of emotional and physical depletion that can lead to mental, respiratory, digestive, and menstrual symptoms.

Heather Preston works as a freelance resource management consultant (a.k.a. "head hunter") for national software firms. Before going freelance she directed the human resources division of a large computer corporation. When the company had to downsize its staff, she was involved in helping the people she had fired to find new employment, and she spent a lot of time holding their hands in the interim. She left that job after five years, because she found herself emotionally depleted from helping everyone else. Now that she's self-employed she can better regulate her professional output. She has, however, taken on the position of treasurer and fundraiser for her choral society and still spends a lot of telephone time solving her friends' problems.

The exaggeration of concern and nurturing can also turn inward. The care-giving that characterizes Spleen types can transform into introspection and unhealthy self-absorption. This can develop into fretting

---

tis goes better, my sense of self is better, everything works well.—*Joan Kip*
I began offering acupuncture to a few patients who had problems that my western-type practice could do nothing for. To my total surprise and great joy, these treatments really and truly worked. They worked so well on so many complex and difficult problems, it felt like magic. And it was a type of magic, just like the first time I looked through a microscope and could see a whole world I had never known existed.—*Robert Chase, M.D.*

over minor and major problems and may, in its extreme form, lead to serious obsessive behavior. Excessive pensiveness and brooding on ideas and emotions can, in turn, weaken Spleen Qi in its role of supervising thought and mental focus, as can excessive study and memorization. People with depleted Spleen Qi look to be nurtured, but seem to never receive enough. They constantly need to tell others about their problems. Such disturbances in Spleen Qi can be described as being ungrounded, unfocused in life, unable to concentrate on the task at hand. We have all encountered such people during their needy periods, and we recall how difficult it is to truly help them with consolation or advice.

When Spleen Qi is full and healthy, Nurture/Duty types possess extraordinary stamina, even a fierce energy in pursuit of duty or pleasure and gratification. When Spleen Qi is less vital, though, habits of excess eating or indulging can take over. With weakened Spleen Qi, these types can become lazy and sedentary, for example, getting up late, lying in bed or napping at any time of the day, only enjoying the moment. Not generally athletically inclined, Nurture/Duty types easily lose the discipline it takes to exercise and maintain a healthy body. Even the joyfulness of the bon vivant can be cyclical. The appealing and entertaining charmer at the cocktail party might exhibit a foul-tempered irritability the next day. He is at all times obsessive about his bowel habits and will experience bowel irritability during times of pressure.

Nurture/Duty people with a Lung-Intestine-Metal makeup can find that their sense of duty bears a quality of self-criticism, augmented because their goals of perfection are impossible to achieve. They can be rigid and judgmental of others to an unpleasant extreme. Their ability to exercise judgment and make decisions in the workplace can escalate to a desire to control everything they do and all those around them. Instead

---

The first night was a bloody miracle. I just slept and slept. I hadn't slept for months. You saved my life in the middle of those crises.—*Joan Kip*

I have had some spectacular on-the-table experiences: goopy ears drying up, chest releasing congestion, and sinuses draining. Acupuncture has taken me from a sense of ill-being to a point where my body is in charge again. That is the most remarkable effect I have had. It takes me from being sick at one moment to being well, usually an

of having an infectious joy in life and pleasure, Lung types can fall into sadness and peevish bad moods. Their voices become tinged with tones of grief and melancholy. They share the ritual of bowel movements and cyclical mood patterns with their bon vivant Earth partners, but with a greater tendency to disabling depression.

Mary Wilson is especially susceptible to respiratory infections in late autumn and early winter. She must pay special attention to maintaining her health through regular rest and exercise. If she falls ill, she also falls into a self-critical fatigued state that can be colored with mild depression. She always completes projects out of a sense of duty, even if the activities are draining her while she is ill. If, for example, she is not punctual with her home-baked birthday and Christmas goodies for my office staff, she is genuinely upset and apologizes for her tardiness.

Functional and Organic Pathology of the Spleen

When the Spleen is unable to convert solid and liquid nourishment into useful energy and move it to the Lungs for circulation, a general feeling of lassitude, forgetfulness, stiffness, and fatigue will occur. This can be coupled with a sallow or pasty complexion and pale, dry lips. If the crucial functions of transforming and transporting food and fluid are disturbed, digestive symptoms arise: loss of appetite; a sour taste; heartburn; hiccups or burping; nausea or vomiting; stomach irritation; a sense of fullness or bloating in the abdomen; gas and diarrhea or constipation; as well as difficulty in losing or maintaining weight.

In conventional medicine we lack specific diagnoses for these undifferentiated symptoms, so we call them "functional" problems. We know that something is not functioning correctly, but we cannot measure

---

overnight experience. My problems are not fixed, but I feel like I've taken a turn for the better, and that it has lasted.—*Mary Wilson*

The acupuncture relieved the pressure and tension in my neck muscles that I had since the surgery many years ago. It worked right away, even with the first treatment. Since then, every treatment has relieved tension and pain in my neck and back. When we first started I couldn't turn my neck to 45° in either direction. Now I can turn

or define any recognized disease. Functional symptoms, if unacknowl-edged and untreated over a period of time, can develop into true organ pathology. Digestive tract disturbances, when they evolve from func-tional into more serious pathology, finally receive official medical names: obesity, gastro-esophageal reflux disease (GERD), peptic ulcer disease (PUD), irritable bowel syndrome (IBS), and the inflammatory bowel diseases (Crohn's disease and ulcerative colitis). These gastro-intestinal disturbances occur most commonly in people with Nurture/Duty biopsychotypes.

Heather Preston, solidly Spleen-Earth, gains weight easily when she overeats or neglects her exercise. She lost the weight she gained during her final year at the computer company, and took great pride in the control she regained over her eating habits when she started to work for herself. Within six months, though, she had succumbed to the increased pressure from her successful consulting business and started to regain the lost weight. She also developed irritable bowel symptoms. A crash diet of salads and vegetable juice failed to restore mastery of her weight. A year after going into solo practice she was in an unhappy state: obsessed with work yet not working effectively, lacking the energy to exercise, and lacking the discipline to diet. She looked heavy and swollen and complained of uncomfortable heaviness in her thighs and aching in her ankles. She became uncharacter-istically resistant to my recommendations that she rearrange her work habits and obligations to include exercise. She refused to discuss her weight or listen to diet recommendations. Here, Heather displayed physical and psychological manifestations of "dampness," caused by depleted Spleen energy.

90° in both directions. I could not lift my right arm above my head. Now I work twelve hours a day using my arms and shoulders and neck, without pain. If the pain returns, I make an appointment to have acupuncture, and the pain gets under control again.—*Audrose Calhoun*
The needles certainly sped up my recovery after surgery. When I had the bladder repair you needled the incision when I got out of the hospital. I've never seen any-

Dampness

In the Chinese medical tradition the general symptoms of deficient Spleen activity are caused by an internal state of dampness. This is an extremely common condition in our modern world with our intense activity and pressure, our frequent carelessmess regarding the quality of our food, and the hurried conditions under which we eat our meals. Dampness is most often caused by eating excess quantities of what are considered to be cold- and damp-producing foods, which create sluggishness and stagnation in the digestive process. A short list of these foods includes raw salads and fruits, uncooked vegetables, vegetable and fruit juices, iced drinks and cold desserts, dairy products, wheat products, and refined sugars. All of these are popular items for the busy person. Eating at irregular times, inadequate or excessive eating, eating quickly, working during lunch, even watching television during meals are co-conspirators in developing dampness in the digestive tract.

Prolonged exposure to damp climates such as foggy mountain or seaside regions, damp houses, sitting or working on damp surfaces, wearing damp clothing after swimming or exercising, or suffering any protracted disease can also cause dampness. So can chronic worry or obsessive thinking – about self, life situations, or others – or depression. The most important causes, however, are cold- and damp-producing foods and irregular eating habits, together with a constitutional weakness in this domain. Those of other constitutions might never develop symptoms of dampness from a regular diet of cold foods and drinks, to the envy of their Nurture/Duty friends and colleagues.

---

thing heal so fast. Flat, no raised scar tissue, no pain at the incision.—*Mary Wilson*
When I had surgery on my wrist you told me to come by the office soon after the operation. I was kicked out immediately following the procedure, even after a general anesthetic. My husband brought me straight to your office and dragged me to the table. You put in some needles and I became clear, alert, and energized within five minutes. This impressed

The state of dampness interferes not only with the digestive activities of the Spleen, but also with its other functions. For example, the Spleen's responsibility to keep blood in the vessels is also important. Failure in this function results in visible surface capillaries, easy bruising, varicose veins, hemorrhoids, and heavy or lengthy menstrual periods. Fluid retention manifests as swelling or edema in the face, abdomen, or ankles. When the Spleen fails to adequately nourish and control the muscles, especially in the extremities, one experiences weariness and weakness in the muscles and cold and heaviness in the limbs. General complaints of heaviness in the arms, chest, abdomen, pelvis, or thighs derive from this aspect of Spleen's weakness.

Spleen also plays a critical role in supervising menstruation, fertility, pregnancy, and recovery after childbirth. Of all life functions, childbirth is the most demanding and depleting of Spleen's vitality. Without a fully functioning Spleen (remember, we're talking about Spleen function, not about the western spleen organ) and regular, healthy periods, conceiving and maintaining pregnancies can become difficult. After delivery, women risk not returning to their pre-pregnancy state of energy, weight, health, emotional stability, or mental clarity, if Spleen Qi is not restored. They are especially susceptible to problems of varicosities, hemorrhoids, and retained fluid. Pregnancy and delivery challenge another important Spleen function, that of holding organs in their proper place. Weakened Spleen Qi and the resulting dampness in the body tissue can cause other organs to lose their support. The bladder, uterus, vagina, and rectum can all drop, or prolapse, later in life, especially after childbirth or menopause.

---

even my husband, who had been skeptical. And, I never had any pain from the surgery.—*Elena Verde*

I was under general anesthesia for a five-hour surgery, and the next day the surgeon kept coming into my room to see if I was breathing properly. I wasn't. It felt like I was trying to suck air through a mass of wet cobwebs, and was just able to get the

Mary Ellen Hannibal is a disciplined and articulate writer and editor. She is also an attentive mother. At age thirty-five she explained that she had not regained her strength and stamina since the birth of her daughter:

I feel like I am running on empty, that I don't have the reserves with which to go about my daily life. I work part time and have a four-year-old. It takes everything I have just to keep moving.

This is a state of depleted Spleen Qi. Over the course of a year we had a dozen acupuncture sessions, and I added a homeopathic remedy into her treatment. Today she has a second child, feels healthy and energetic, and is able to balance family and work while maintaining her own well-being.

Longstanding dampness from poor eating habits, from a constitutional weakness in the Nurture/Duty terrain, from prolonged worry, chronic illness, maternity, or aging creates a body that feels and looks heavy. The generalized sluggish movement of energy and blood creates doughiness and edema in the tissue. This state of stagnant circulation can settle in an area and cause oppression in the chest, heaviness in the abdomen, or congestion in the pelvis. It can result in chronic mucus in the sinuses, nose, and lungs, and chronic vaginal discharge. As dampness stagnates it can congeal into nodules just under the skin. These can appear around painful joints or as tissue masses such as fibrocystic breast tissue and uterine fibroid tumors.

I saw **Heather Preston** at a social function two years after she interrupted her series of acupuncture treatments. She was even more obese than the last time I had seen her professionally. We talked briefly about her year-long battle with irregular periods and pelvic fullness, which had

---

most shallow of breaths. Then you put one needle in my chest, and even before your hand left the needle everything kicked in and I took a huge deep wonderful breath. I wouldn't have believed it possible if it hadn't happened to me.—*Penny Sinclair*
My daughter was having a hard time. The third baby was due on Monday but was positioned with the head down but the face up. She did not want another Caesarian. She sat in your waiting room with needles in her toes and jumper cables attached. She

recently been diagnosed as massive uterine fibroids. She announced that she was shopping for a gynecologist who would remove the fibroids without requiring that she lose weight before surgery.

Functional and Organic Pathology of the Lung

The quality of Lung Qi is determined by its innate strength plus the quantity of Spleen Qi contributed by the digestive process. Early manifestations of weak Lung Qi can include frequent sighing, breathlessness, and skin problems. (Remember, skin is considered the third lung.) Dampness from deficient Stomach and Spleen Qi can spread into the Lung territory as well. Signs of Lung dampness include frequent head and chest colds, sinusitis, laryngitis, bronchitis, asthma, and emphysema. Clogged nasal passages, coughing, and excess mucus production are all conditions of Lung dampness.

Because Lung connects with the outside world when we breathe in air, it is vulnerable to inhaled irritants as well as to extremes of weather. Strong Lung Qi is required to defend the body against illness from climate, pollution, or microbes inhaled into its tissue. Strong Lung Qi is also needed to move protective energy to the zone of surface channels in the skin and outer muscle layer, which serve as a shield between the external environment and the inside of the body.

The role of protective energy in maintaining the body's good health cannot be overemphasized. The Chinese classics describe a variety of external conditions as potentially damaging to internal organs. For example, Spleen function is most susceptible to external extremes of dampness, the Liver function to wind, the Kidney to cold, the Heart

---

felt the baby turning, and the obstetrician confirmed it by a sonogram. She went on to a normal birth. An acupuncture miracle!—*Mary Wilson*

The most gratifying effect I have ever gotten was when you saved my legs. The femoral arteries were occluded beyond the reach of arteroplasty, beyond the reach of balloon or surgery. You relieved the pain in my feet, which hurt badly all the time, and with each treatment I was able to walk farther. I was able to fly in comfort after three

to heat, and the Lung to dryness. This is not to say that an extreme external condition will affect only the organ of susceptibility or that external conditions will always affect that organ. Rather, it means that if the body's protective energy is not robust, one of these external conditions could penetrate the body and lodge in an organ where it can cause trouble. Each organ has one special vulnerability, but its disturbances are not necessarily caused by just one external condition.

The Lung is susceptible to dryness on the outside and inside of the body. Just as a dry desert climate is not necessarily the best environment for someone with deficient Lung Qi, Lung Qi weakness from unhealthy eating, worry, depression, menopause, age, or chronic illness can create symptoms of dryness, including dry lips and mouth, hoarse voice, dry cough, and constipation.

The Lung is often the first organ to show the symptoms of an invasion of wind-cold or wind-heat. These descriptive terms can be taken literally to mean an exposure to wind or a draft, or as a metaphor that explains that wind symptoms in the body move quickly from one place to another. Wind-cold appears as muscle aches, stuffy nose, itchy throat, coughing, and feeling cold, in rapid succession – what we call a common cold. Wind-heat describes a cold that goes deeper into the body, takes longer to resolve, and appears as headaches, body aches, sweating, fever, sore throat, and yellow mucus.

Lung Qi is also involved in circulating body fluids to the skin, facilitating the fluid and temperature equilibration that occurs through sweating. Because the skin is within the Lung sphere of influence, deficient Lung energy can result in too much or too little sweating and lowered resistance. Other symptoms of Lung's failure to manage

---

months, and I now use the treadmill in short spurts every day.—*Bill Kane*
Patients not only accept the acupuncture paradigm, but actively seek those techniques and approaches that seem to strike a common, familiar chord, reuniting the myriad parts of the whole which scientific medicine has gone to such great pains to fragment. Many of my patients are hungry for an explanation for their lack of wellness. They sense a need for wholeness to their lives, and, having failed to find relief from tablets

fluids are dry or wrinkled skin and congestion in the upper body. Bad complexion and skin eruptions in general also suggest a weakness in Lung energy.

Remember that among her collection of weak Lung Qi problems, **Mary Wilson** is persistently bothered by acne on her face, chest, and back, although she is now in her seventies. I always reassure her that she is in better health with a few flaring acne spots than having the inflammation in her lungs.

Many Lung-Metal types have a history of childhood allergies, eczema, frequent respiratory infections, or asthma, acne as an adolescent, and as an adult these may continue or evolve into psoriasis or other skin problems. There is commonly a family history of respiratory frailty, emphysema, or tuberculosis. Respiratory infections easily turn to wheezing. Curiously, the Lung deficient patient may smoke or have smoked cigarettes, even as an adult fully informed of the health dangers of this habit. Evidently the Lung interprets the heat and stimulation of the inhaled smoke as a tonification of its weakness; hence, the body craves the effect. While the heat may feel therapeutic, nicotine addiction and tissue damage from heat and smoke can be, as we know, catastrophic. This paradox recalls the abuse of alcohol and caffeine sometime seen in people with Liver Qi problems.

Mitchell Bernstein is a fifty-six year-old attorney who had recurrent colds and bronchitis as a kid. As an intellectually driven and disciplined adolescent he developed bowel symptoms of bloating, pain, constipation, and diarrhea. By the age of thirty he had full-blown ulcerative colitis. After fifteen years of using corticosteroids to suppress the inflammation in his

---

and technology, are anxious to try something new.—*Michael Acord, M.D.*
The idealized future is one that integrates the two traditions and creates a language wherein one can directly communicate in both directions. One of the great strengths of acupuncture is that it does not divide up body, mind, and spirit. I think acupuncture philosophy and treatment will instigate further developments in the west by

colon, he finally required a colectomy to "resolve" the colitis. The surgery did not, however, restore him to full and robust health. He came to see me with a ten-year history of chronic bronchitis and years of constant antibiotic use. He continued to smoke cigarettes during the first five years of this condition.

Mitchell's biopsychotype is strongly weighted in the Nurture/Duty – Metal arena. His good intellect and memory, coupled with strong discipline, got him into law school. As an attorney he sought noble pursuits, working with non-profit organizations throughout his career. He has followed a devotional spiritual discipline for several decades and helps with legal matters that involve the local ashram as well as the construction of a hospital in India. These aspects of his personality illustrate strong Nurture/Duty. His childhood bronchitis reflects a weakness, probably inherited, in Lung Qi. During his adolescence, the Intestine (the other Metal organ) was affected by his inherited energetic weakness, and his symptoms shifted to the digestive system.

When the Intestine did not recover from its disease and was removed, the weakness intrinsic in Nurture/Duty-Metal returned to the Lung to create the bronchitis anew. Mitchell described himself as usually being upbeat and positive, but the year before seeing me he had slipped into mild depression because of the concern for his health. We worked on his Lung vitality, his protective energy, and his digestive process with acupuncture, then added Chinese herbal formulas to reinforce the acupuncture treatments. After six months of treatments every two weeks, his lungs stabilized without antibiotics, and his overall vitality returned. He now takes a low-dose herbal regimen and comes in for tune-up acupuncture treatments before each change of season, thereby maintaining his stamina and good Lung Qi even while traveling extensively for work or with his spiritual teacher.

those who are not uncomfortable with its foreign nature and different language.—*John Giusto, M.D.*

My years of education and medical training had made me a Cartesian, a linear thinker constantly seeking cause-effect relationships. Early in my acupuncture training I was compelled to think about patterns and relationships, associating symptoms with biopsychotypes, or more complex five phases correspondences. At times I felt uneasy

I've completed the description of two biopsychotypes: Vision/ Action and Nurture/Duty. By now, you may have some sense of how much Vision/Action and Nurture/Duty contribute to your unique constitution. In the next chapter, I finish the series by examining the realm of Will/Spirit. If you are eager to read what you can do to gain best value from your Nurture/Duty constitution, you may read Chapter 10 now, even before exploring the Will/Spirit biopsychotype. If the characteristics and symptoms of these first two biopsychotypes are starting to blur in your memory, you may refer to Appendix I for simplified summaries of the types, rather than rereading the chapters.

and confused, but I hung in, anticipating some revelation that would ease my discomfort. It did not come until months after the course's end, when gradually my schizoid medical thinking became more facile, able to switch easily between my allopathic thinking and acupuncture thinking and back again. Then, as I practiced acupuncture more, the experience became more like viewing an Escher painting, able to see first the fishes, then the rabbits; first the causal, then the pattern. I realized I had finally accomplished the final step of integrating the new discipline with the old, and I became proficient in Escherian switching.—*Allen McDaniels, M.D.*

As I began to take expanded acupuncture-style histories with an open demeanor, I noticed that patients often presented unusual symptoms, ones that might be dismissed as psychosomatic or hypochondriacal. If I teased out more from the history and formatted it into an acupuncture template, and treated the subcircuit of the predominant symptom, lo and

CHAPTER 7

WILL/SPIRIT BIOPSYCHOTYPE

Jim Barmakian, Renee Carter's fiancé, showed his forthright and direct demeanor when he spoke out at her first appointment. Jim embodies the signature qualities of the Will/Spirit biopsychotype. He is clear thinking and motivated, direct in his expression, and hard-working, and he expects to be in command of his life and activities. He also has a special vulnerability to low back pain. Being his weak physical link, it will typically flare when he's feeling the pressures of change or losing control.

A year after he married Renee, Jim came to the office as a patient. He was having trouble getting rid of a backache that started after a round of golf with his father. The pain was primarily on the left side of his lower back, but occasionally it shot into the buttock and back of his leg, all the way down to his little toe. When the pain was acting up, Jim had trouble concentrating on his work and getting good sleep. While polite, Jim was quietly impatient to finish talking and get on with the treatment. He knew acupuncture's potential from having watched Renee's response, and he urgently wanted his pain to go away.

Jim is an attorney; he was successful early in his career by guiding a software company to its initial public offering. That achievement gave him the confidence to launch his own venture capital endeavor that, unfortunately, was not moving in the direction he wanted. During the round of golf, Jim was discussing with his father the possibility of merging his new operation into his father's established venture capital firm.

Water and Fire

As with Vision/Action and Nurture/Duty, there are two sides to Will/Spirit. Looking at the elements that give the poetic qualities to this biopsychotype, we see that the Will/Spirit terrain combines the adaptability

---

behold, very often the other so-called psychosomatic symptoms would resolve with the treatment as well. Thus I became aware of what a powerful tool acupuncture is for diagnosis and treatment.—*Patrick Magovern, M.B.B.S.*
After thirty-six years as a surgeon I learned that I can serve my patients better by simply listening, questioning, and palpating them at tender points in their tissues. A thin, tiny needle is the communicating instrument between me and them.—*Hiroshi Nakazawa, M.D.*

of Water with the spark and passion of Fire. (We encountered Fire earlier in Chapter 5 in its affiliation with Master of the Heart and Triple Heater.) At first thought, Water and Fire seem a strangely incompatible combination of characteristics in the same biopsychotype. The two other element pairings (Wood and Fire, Earth and Metal) are less strikingly extreme than this one and make sense when we understand the influences of the organs. As unlikely as it may first seem, the linking together of Water and Fire makes sense as well.

Water is essential for life; it makes up much of the body's volume. Water as an element is the image for movement and change: springs, flowing streams, waterfalls, and oceans. It adapts to fill any container; it refreshes and invigorates; it can be placid or forceful; it bathes and cleanses and nourishes. The person with predominant Water qualities can be quiet and adaptable or can, on occasion, be forceful and clearly noticed. But he is always present and willing to contribute. The season associated with Water is winter, the season of cold and conservation of effort.

The image of *Fire* embodies the sun, blazing light and heat, vitality and warmth, rising energy, and mental brilliance. The sun gives life, warms and nourishes, and is the constant core of energy in our solar system. Fire connotes heating and circulation, generating and maintaining physical and emotional warmth, enthusiasm, and creativity. The season associated with Fire is summer, the season of growth and maturation.

When combined in a balanced Will/Spirit person, Water and Fire qualities are integrated and collaborating. Water and its associated organ, the Kidney, bring will and power to the individual. Fire

---

Learning and practicing acupuncture has made me more perceptive, more thoughtful, a better listener, and has deepened my understanding of people. It has made me a more compassionate person and a better physician.—*Marshall Sager, D.O.*
I discovered that, although acupuncture was not always the cure, the increased amount of time it gave me to sit with patients, hear their stories, and really bear witness to their problems was a healing modality in and of itself. Although I explained to these

and its associated organ, the Heart, bring spirit and passion. Together Water and Fire create and maintain the impulses of self-direction and creativity. If you are a predominantly Will/Spirit person, you are level-headed, intellectually lively, willful, and decisive. You are comfortable being a leader, and in this role you are balanced and effective. You are usually healthy and assume you can do whatever you set your mind to do. You automatically find yourself the clear-thinking motivator in your organization, providing structure and direction and sparking enthusiasm in those around you.

Young **Jim Barmakian** certainly shows these qualities in his makeup. At twenty-nine, his Fire qualities are dominant in his personality and life choices. This balance, however, is always subject to change as life unfolds.

You met **Johnny Maddox** in Chapter 4. He is a former truck driver now in his late seventies, who has been seeing me since he was fifty-five for acupuncture management of the pain and limitations created by spinal stenosis, a crippling problem in his vertebral column. Despite his evolving physical discomfort, he has always been a natural leader. In high school he was student body president and captain of the football team, and he organized his fiftieth class reunion. He has always been motivated to excel in his work and take advantage of the opportunities life presents him. He still owns and supervises his own transmission repair business.

He started life with more Fire than Water, but since his third decade the Water qualities have gained the upper hand. John's Will/Spirit constitution allows him to live day-to-day with the inconvenience of constant pain, without falling into depression or despair. His "Grit, God, and Gumption!"

---

patients that I was not their primary care practitioner, many of them told me that I was really much more their personal physician than were their actual primary care doctors, who could spend only five or ten minutes a visit with them.—*Brian Bouch, M.D.*

If there are providers in a practice who can perform acupuncture, this will help many people get better without costly procedures or poorly justified surgeries. It will directly affect modern medicine. Acupuncture has its greatest application as the first

motto manifests in his unconquerable spirit and his will to survive with dignity. His Will allows him to accommodate to his limitations and create a daily routine that includes work, reading, and co-chairing a support group for others who suffer from chronic pain.

Water can be still and deep or powerful and dynamic. Water vitality shows as strength in dealing with challenges, a strength that is not ostentatious, but quiet and internal. People with an abundance of Water energy gain respect as reliable members of the team, who are rarely outspoken and do not draw attention to themselves. They appear calm, are quiet, and do not make conversation easily. They will speak out, however, when they deem it necessary to do so.

On the other hand, Fire brings to mind excitement and creativity. People with generous Fire qualities like to be seen and heard, and they bring joy and laughter to those around them. They make quick emotional connections with others and are warm, open, and direct in relationships. Fire types are expansive, talkative, seductive, and happy to be alive. The quality of Fire is associated with ideas and their expression through words. Fire types can have insightful intellects that allow them to quickly comprehend complex situations and act confidently and creatively. The intimate side of a Fire person is empathetic, sensitive, and intuitive.

You also met **Julie Mendosa** in Chapter 4. Julie grew up in a California Mexican family of modest means, and, thanks to her determination and entrepreneurial drive, she created a successful business supplies enterprise. Julie is attractive, warm, fast-talking, and persuasive. She thinks even faster than she talks and can maneuver a sales interview or social encounter in any direction she desires. She can solve office organization and operation

---

step in dealing with musculoskeletal pain and psychosomatic problems. For many people it may be the best choice and the only approach necessary.—*Kirk Pappas, M.D.* I believe that, much more than simply looking at acupuncture as an alternative technique, we must look at these complementary approaches as a new paradigm for viewing health and illness, and delivering health care. What can we distill from acupuncture that will help us understand ourselves and our patients? Do we really need a scientific

problems while selling indispensable office supplies to clients who, before her visit, might not have known that the products were indispensable. She can pump up her Fire for any encounter, but acknowledges that she also values her private time, and being quietly alone with her husband.

Functions and Influences of the Kidney

Kidney is associated with Water in the body's ecology. Just as Water is the indispensable foundation of the body's anatomy, physiology, and biochemistry, so Qi from the Kidney is the indispensable energy in the body. Kidney energy brings with it a special life-driving quality called "essence." The traditional texts refer to Kidney as the "root of life," because it is responsible for the core life functions of reproduction and growth and for animating the Qi in all organs.

Kidney's sphere of influence includes personal, professional, and sexual drive. Kidney supervises the bones and teeth, ears, the sense of hearing, and balance. The quality of Kidney energy is reflected in the moistness and strength of head hair (not body hair). Kidney and Water are associated with the season of winter, dark blue or black colors, and salty flavors. In acupuncture physiology, just as in conventional physiology, Kidney and Bladder work together to create, store, and excrete urine, and thus rid the body of impure and excess fluids.

In its role of supervising bones and bone marrow, Kidney is responsible for joints and flexibility. Teeth are also bone and are therefore ruled by Kidney. If Kidney energy is strong, the bones will be strong and the teeth firm. The importance of the spinal column and the skeletal structure reaffirms the critical importance of Kidney energy in

---

model to understand Qi, or does acupuncture, and the other forms of energy medicine, exist outside this model that we have so obediently followed for the last 150 years?— *Todd Lininger, M.D.*

There are many parallels between osteopathic manipulative medicine and medical acupuncture. The philosophies of the approach to patients are overlapping, and I find the combination of approaches gives me the best results. For example, if I use

maintaining the body's infrastructure. The brain is considered to be the marrow of the skull, thus Kidney also nourishes thinking and concentration and oversees physical movement directed by the brain and central nervous system.

Essence

The Kidney is indispensable in maintaining the body's vitality. Kidney energy nourishes, warms, and activates all the other organs. This critical role is attributed to the Kidney because it stores and distributes life essence. Essence is the condensed and concentrated Qi that we inherit from our parents, our chromosomal charge. It differs from nourishing and protective energy, which are derived from food and air on a daily basis. Essence is the source of life; all organs need essence to survive. Essence is active in growth, development, maturity, and senescence. It reaches its peak at puberty and is vital in the functions of conception, pregnancy, and childbirth. Kidney energy weakens and essence diminishes in old age; the reproductive function declines, and the body and its organs slow down in their activities.

Essence is the hereditary energy that determines our constitutional strength. It is created at the moment of conception, when the male and female reproductive energies merge. It creates the biopsychotype of an individual. Essence works with protective energy to resist illness caused by external climatic and environmental extremes. The quantity and quality of one's essence are fixed and must be preserved by striving for balance in life's activities.

Kidney Qi and essence determine our will power and motivation. Strong essence creates strong will and the ability to focus the mind on our goals. With strong Kidney Qi we are capable of hard work over long

acupuncture first to soften up the contracted muscles in a musculoskeletal pain problem, I can get much further with my osteopathic manipulation. In the end, combining techniques usually means I see a patient less frequently and for a shorter course of therapy than with one approach alone.—*Gary Kaplan, D.O.*

I found that acupuncture works for some things I have, but doesn't work for others. At some point along the line I stopped worrying about how much money I was spending,

periods of time. Essence provides the impulse for sexual expression, for procreation, for continuing the flow of life from one generation to the next. Kidney Qi and essence are also the foundations of mental vigor, the manifestation of which is supervised by the Heart.

Functions and Influences of the Heart

The Heart embodies the qualities of Fire in the body. The active part of the autonomic nervous system (Master of the Heart) also pulls Fire into action by protecting the functions of the Heart, but not to the same extent as Heart itself. The most important energetic function of the Heart is housing the spirit. Its most important physiological functions are pumping blood through the arteries and governing the blood and blood vessels. In traditional texts the Heart is described as the emperor who rules the body in all physical, psychological, and spiritual aspects. Thus, governing blood and housing the spirit encompass the critical responsibilities of the emperor: keeping the constitution strong and inspiring creativity and expression.

Spirit

Essence from the Kidney determines the constitutional vitality of an individual. Spirit from the Heart supplies vigor and strength to the constitution. A strong spirit creates a clear consciousness, creative thinking, good memory, balanced emotions, and good sleep. Spirit allows us to be happy in our emotions, actively engaged in our relationships, and at peace with our place in the universe. When Heart energy is in balance, the spirit is lively, the mind is open, the eyes are clear, and the complexion is bright. We can express ourselves creatively and articulately. Spirit refines and manifests the will and focus created by essence. Heart and Kidney thus complement one another in their energetic functions.

because I was balancing how well I felt against the cost. I just decided that I was going to have a once-a-month tune-up. And I'm glad I made the decision.—*Elena Verde*
I think the insurance companies should take one step further and cover acupuncture for preventive treatments. I know that if I come in every three or four weeks it keeps me away from the more expensive visits to other doctors and procedures. I strongly believe that the insurance companies should sponsor this.—*Julie Mendosa*

Julie Mendosa is our most Fiery patient. Her intense presence – voice, laughter, perfume – makes itself known the moment she enters the office. She brings empathy, direction, and passion to everything she undertakes.

When the energy of the Heart is strong there is abundant blood, the blood vessels are healthy, and the pulse is full and regular. Blood suffuses all the organs and tissues of the body, and its abundance is reflected in a rosy complexion. The Heart creates joy and connectedness among people. The quality of the Heart is also represented in the color, form, and surface of the tongue, especially its tip. The Heart influences speech, which includes laughter as well as articulate verbal expression. The sense of taste is in the Heart's sphere of influence, as are sweating and dreaming. Heart and Fire are also associated with an affinity for red hues, an affection for bitter or roasted flavors, and a strong like – or dislike – of summer and hot weather.

Manifestations of Will/Spirit Disturbances

Three typical disturbance patterns affect persons of predominantly Will/Spirit biopsychotype, depending on the unique mix of Water and Fire they start with.

- The balanced Water-Fire type is vulnerable to backaches (as are the Heart-Fire and Kidney-Water types).
- Heart-Fire types can become excitable and lose focus.
- Kidney-Water energy can become depleted and result in fatigue and pain.

I can't count the number of times I have heard some variation of "I didn't know the military does acupuncture," or "I can't believe they let you do acupuncture in the Army." People forget that many of the medical and technological advances that we take for granted came from military medicine and research. I can usually get people to agree that "If the military is doing it, well, then, it must be okay!"—*Steven Braverman, M.D., Colonel, U.S. Army*

Water and Fire in Equal Measure

The balanced Will/Spirit person is levelheaded, intellectually lively, willful, and decisive, and often holds a leadership position. Someone of this composition is usually confident of his abilities and successful in his endeavors. He often enjoys and can excel at sports. But unlike his Vision/Action counterparts, who cannot be inactive, and who play sports for the love of movement, the Will/Spirit person seeks the intensity of competition. If he is overshadowed in his skill, he wins by will and drive. Interestingly, however, this person is also protective of his personal life and habits and is reluctant to reveal anything about himself that might display flaws or shortcomings in physical health, personal habits, or intellectual accomplishment. He expects perfection from himself and those around him.

Two varieties of disturbance can develop in this person, either a Fire form or a Water form. The *Fire form* typically exaggerates the confidence and authority of the Will/Spirit type and converts them into an imperious, imposing presence, with voice too strong and demeanor too assured. The person in this state tends to dominate in relationships of any nature. He displays unambiguous impatience and arrogance and candidly acknowledges this description as both accurate and justified. As the Fire exaggeration takes over the personality of the balanced Will/Spirit individual, he can easily erupt into anger or become intoxicated with a sense of invincibility and invulnerability. In extreme cases, this can degenerate to extravagant sexual, business, or political indiscretions, insensible to rational guidance.

Immediately after the first treatment I had a sense of well-being, a sense that there is something other than a pill to help keep me well. With the help of the needles, I did it myself! Coming for acupuncture makes the HIV a more palatable malady to deal with. Acupuncture also took care of the pain in my feet coming from the medication. Nobody will be cured of HIV with acupuncture, but it is a method to empower the person to keep himself well by balance and energy.—*Gregory Marshall*

We can all recall a recent American president – intelligent, resourceful, and passionate – whose success and arrogance imbued him with a sense of invulnerability to criticism of his extramarital adventures while in office. This was Fire out of control, impervious to the balancing effects of Water that could constrain and redirect his passion. (We also know that this president later developed physical heart problems that required bypass surgery.)

The *Water form,* on the contrary, experiences a loss of confidence that creates doubts and prevents clear decisions and actions in someone who is usually commanding and assertive. These mental and emotional features are likely to be accompanied by a diminished physical vitality, a sense that the body's stamina can no longer be relied upon to execute the habitual workload and responsibilities. The diminished vitality can be accompanied by touchiness or impatience, disturbed sleep, digestive discomfort or diarrhea, bladder or urinary disorders, and an increasing sensitivity to cold. The Will/Spirit person in this Water state is likely to be psychologically touchy if queried about his health or decisions and, like his Fire counterpart, will be impatient with the inconvenience of illness and the imperfection it implies.

Georgia Quan is a forty-eight-year-old CEO of a trading company dealing with Asian products. She was infected with Lyme disease six months ago while on vacation in New England. Even though it was treated promptly and most of her symptoms resolved, she has "not felt back to par" since the infection. While easy fatigue was among her most bothersome symptoms, she also brought up other problems not immediately connected with Lyme disease: sensitivity to cold weather; diffuse lumbar pain that flares when she travels; feeling more concerned and fearful than she remembers; and an annoying recurrent bladder infection despite a waning of her sexual

---

The back pain didn't change after the first session, but after the third or fourth treatment I began to feel better in general. The pain changed, and mentally I was given a new life, almost like a shot of morphine that eased the pain and picked me up. Not all my pain went away, but it was like being in a dark room and someone snapped the light on. This thorn I'd had since high school, it was not removed, but its quality had been changed. Now I know that I'll feel achy for a day, and then the improvement starts. I

activity. Georgia has always been able to count on her Will/Spirit vitality to do whatever she wants. The Lyme infection pushed her into a state where the Fire edge of her spirit was overcome by Water features, and she did not want to surrender to these changes.

Back Pain

Back pain is the common weak link in balanced Will/Spirit people, whether their disharmonies tend toward the Fire or Water direction. The organs in this energy subcircuit generate and drive our essence and spirit, the psychospiritual infrastructure for our survival and self-expression. On the physical level, Kidney and Heart supervise bones, bone marrow, and blood, the skeletal infrastructure of our bodies. A healthy backbone and nervous system are as critical to our survival and self-expression as are essence and spirit.

The body zone most influenced by the energy pathways of the Will/Spirit organs is the back: from the back of the head and neck to the vertebral column and the muscles running alongside it to the buttocks and back of the legs. The spinal cord, vertebral column, and surrounding muscles enable us to stand upright and move. For people of this biopsychotype, the skeleton is their weak link.

The archetypal Will/Spirit patient comes to the acupuncturist's office seeking treatment for low back pain. He can be either impatient, with very acute spasm and pain (like Jim Barmakian) or irritable with pain that has turned chronic (probably because he didn't want to be inconvenienced by seeking treatment earlier). He reluctantly acknowledges that stresses and worries provoke and aggravate the spasm. He answers the interview questions with clarity and directness but is politely impatient

---

can count on it.—*Johnny Maddox*
Acupuncture improved the overall quality of my life after the surgery and radiation, when I was into a mood of "It's not going to get any better." Now I can count on doing things that I could do before surgery. In that respect it improved my attitude and gave me a much better life to look forward to. And you can't ask for much more than that.— *Audrose Calhoun*

with questions that don't seem to him to be relevant to the immediate problem. If this is a second or third episode of low back pain, he grudgingly accepts that it is a recurrent pattern linked to age, body type, and stress.

Back pain is often the only thing that ever goes wrong with the person of integrated Will/Spirit biopsychotype. The lower back is by far the most common location of pain, but it can occur anywhere along the vertebral column from neck to sacrum, with or without pain radiating into the arms or legs. The back pain is caused by the vertebrae and disks putting unusual torsion on the nerves exiting from the spine. It is as commonly precipitated by tension and fatigue as by strain or deterioration of the vertebrae. This mechanism of pain is different from that of the Vision/Action types, where the muscles are chronically irritable in and of themselves, and can become inflamed and contracted without being triggered from the vertebral column or nerve irritation. Backache in a Will/Fire person can be Fire in nature, that is, acute, spastic, and very painful with movement; or it can be Water in nature, the persistent ache of a chronic or recurrent problem.

Back pain is not unique to Will/Spirit biopsychotypes; it occurs in people of all biopsychotypes who have deterioration of the spine. If the backache becomes chronic, its very duration creates fatigue and Kidney depletion. The will diminishes, because the restrictions in activity also restrict one's ambition and goals, and the spirit becomes flat with the disappointment of chronic pain. This is the weak link especially of the balanced Will/Spirit constitution.

Having acupuncture is like hitting the reset button on the computer. Suddenly I have all my RAM back.—*Linda Sheldon*
Acupuncture hasn't cured me, but it's given me great relief. Now when I'm feeling really bad and that old sensation is there again, with just one treatment it's gone, just that quick. Acupuncture doesn't only take away the pain, it takes away the tiredness that comes from being in pain all the time. I think I've had acupuncture on all parts of my body. In my

Exaggerations in Heart–Fire

People endowed with abundant Heart energy and generous Fire in their personalities are passionate, have bright complexions and are unreservedly noisy merrymakers and good party guests. They are intense in their presence, and they like to be seen. Women wear brilliant clothing and sparkling jewels and bangles. Clothing and underwear are frequently reds and pinks. Usually Fire types prefer warm weather to cool, but they are not uncomfortable in cold. They perspire easily and become irritable on hot days.

People in the Heart zone of the Will/Spirit spectrum are quick in everything, and even appear frenzied to those who don't share Fire characteristics. They eat quickly, talk quickly, walk quickly, and get through their work quickly. Someone with Fire energy in excess can make those around him feel uncomfortable because of his intensity. He can be amusing as the life of the party, but he might continue telling jokes and dominating the situation when it's no longer appropriate. His laughter might grow too loud or last too long. Or he might have a short temper and explode quickly when someone's not living up to his expectations.

The typical Heart excess patient comes to see the acupuncturist with complaints of agitation, insomnia, and difficulty calming down. He wants to take the nervous edge off his agitated state, but he does not want to be tranquilized. He enjoys the intensity of his life and uses his passion in creative work and living. He reacts to stress and frustration with abrupt outbursts of anger. His work colleagues have learned to let him blow off steam occasionally, because he does not hold on to the anger once he's calmed down, and he is very energetic and productive at work. This is Fire in action and the spirit of Heart expressing itself.

---

daily function my body and my mental state are much better because of not taking the drugs for the pain. I've had such a better outlook on my life, on dealing with problems, on handling situations. I'm doing things I would never have dared to try before.—*Mary Johnson*

I think that the cone of moxa that you lit atop the heap of salt you put in my belly button is the most outrageous thing you have ever done to me! But it cured my cramps

Julie Mendosa is exuberant, intense, emotionally expressive, and impossible to ignore:

> *I've always had an exuberance. When I wake up in the mornings, I just want to put on my black seamed stockings and go out and be Me. Mondays are not an issue for me. It's an opportunity to do it again this week, an opportunity to do it better. My exuberance used to get me into situations when I just didn't think much before I spoke or acted. When I was younger, I'd get into trouble because of my wanting to experience things from my toes to my ears.*
>
> *Even now that I'm over forty and am over forty pounds heavier than I was, I've never had my fire put out. When there is something on my mind that's nagging me, I talk myself through it, address the situation, make a plan. I'll create a solution to the problem, and then I just get back on track. I might get angry if somebody's being stupid, but after I've blown off the steam it's all over. I don't stew overnight, and I don't hold grudges.*

Fire out of control leads to restlessness and distraction, difficulty falling asleep, sleep disturbed by dreams, or nighttime wakeful periods of full mental clarity. These more debilitating symptoms can be induced by the intensity with which a Fire type leads his excessively busy life, and be further exacerbated by long periods of stress and high performance. The energy drain from a high-intensity lifestyle depletes the Kidney energy in the biopsychotype equation. In acupuncture terms, Water deficiency fails to keep the Fire of the personality in check. In this situation, ever more intense Fire qualities emerge. If left unchecked, overwhelming Fire can cause psychological and physical collapse or true heart problems.

---

and diarrhea, thank you very much.—*Mary Wilson*
In the practice of acupuncture, a physician evaluates each patient's patterns and creates unique treatment plans. This process is not at all static. It is alive, waiting to be shaped by the practitioner and the patient. In this approach a patient is no longer a statistic; rather, an individual.—*John Foxen, M.D.*
The needles are not going to do for me what my body can't muster itself to do, but

Men and women living in the extreme Fire state of this biopsychotype tend toward exhibitionism and psychological instability and can live in a perpetual romance or psychodrama. Sexual hyperactivity is a common characteristic. Very exaggerated forms will manifest in irrational or hysterical states. The cardiac symptoms can be sharp chest pain or an intense pounding in the chest, rapid heartbeat, restlessness, and dizziness. These symptoms do not necessarily result in true cardiac crisis, although a thorough cardiac evaluation is appropriate at the onset of this state.

The Heart-Fire type can also develop into a state of combined Heart and Kidney depletion. This might be his innate condition or the condition that his Fiery lifestyle led to as he depleted both Heart and Kidney energy. Early symptoms of this condition include an abruptly-appearing fatigue alternating with swings of nervousness. Refreshing sleep is difficult to achieve, and cold feet are the rule. This person feels listless and uninspired and experiences little joy in life. When in this state, the depleted Heart-Fire person can develop true cardiac pathology. In contrast to the exuberant Heart types, those with deficient Heart energy lack emotional force and physical strength. Instead of a rosy face, the complexion turns dull or bluish, the lips pale, and the personality falls flat and colorless.

When **Melina Farandouri** first came to me she was in full Fire mode: red-lipsticked, vital, humorous, talking quickly, exuding heat. She presented herself as being capable in each of her roles: wife, supermom, full-time office manager, daughter, and daughter-in-law. She complained of insomnia accompanied by a pounding heart that got worse around midnight, and a rapid heartbeat at work on days when job demands intensified. The acupuncture calmed her symptoms, but, rather than scheduling more time

---

they will enhance whatever vitality I have. For years I had a cycle of feeling better, then feeling worse, then changing medications and accepting feeling lousy. Now I know that I can trust the acupuncture to help me out, that I don't have to fall apart, that I have a way out. This is very important for my sense of confidence, of being in charge, of not letting the disorder take over me.—*Mary Wilson*

Medical acupuncture, as practiced by well-trained practitioners, taught by enlight-

for herself, she dug in even more passionately at work. Within six months she returned, burned out, and took off a month to recover at home. Her Fire had depleted itself and was replaced by a Water state. She recovered, then went through another cycle of intensifying her activities, and crashed again.

Following the second physical and psychological collapse, she developed a sequence of heart symptoms that were difficult for the cardiologists to diagnose. They tested her for abnormalities in her thyroid and adrenal glands, and they implanted a pacemaker, which didn't seem to make any difference to her symptoms. It took several years and many visits for specialists to finally arrive at a conclusive diagnosis and for her to attain a more stable cardiac status. Her personality now is still scintillating with the original Fire, but she has achieved an integration between her psyche and soma that reflects a hard-earned respect for Water as well.

Exaggerations in Kidney–Water

Kidney energy and essence serve as the pilot light for energy production in all the organs, and thus good Kidney energy is crucial to maintain the internal warmth and vitality of the body. Unlike Heart-Fire problems, Kidney-Water problems stem from depleted energy, rather than excess energy. Deficiency in Kidney Qi can be inherited from parents or acquired from childhood or adult illnesses and lifestyle, or simply evolve as a feature of advancing age. Each person's constitutional composition and strength depend on the quality and strength of his or her parents' essences. If these essences are weak at the time of conception – because of age, or fatigue, or inherited or acquired Kidney weakness – the Kidney strength of the child will not be robust.

---

ened teachers in medical schools, and resting on a foundation of solid research can be the model for a revolution in medicine. The revolution will provide the consumers of medical services with an expanded menu of choices to enhance health and treat disease. But the public must demand access to this expanded menu, and insist that it be provided by competent practitioners with good credentials.—*Allen McDaniels, M.D.*
Acupuncture treatments normalize people. It gets them to lie down for a half-hour or

A child born to parents deficient in Kidney energy is likely to have frequent bouts of flu and repeated throat, ear, and respiratory infections in early years. This occurs because essence is not contributing to the defensive work of protective energy, the acupuncture equivalent of the immune system. The child might not display the same fearless curiosity and physical stamina as his playmates, and can develop a somewhat reticent and awkward personality.

Children who are not innately deficient in Kidney energy can lose Kidney vitality if in childhood they frequently experience infections or more pernicious diseases, or suffer from malnutrition or prolonged periods of physical or emotional deprivation. Children whose essence is not strong – by inheritance or by illness –can suffer retardation of their growth and mental development and start puberty and menses later than their peers. They may appear withdrawn, insecure, and easily panicked. They have a lifetime responsibility to nurture and protect their Kidney vitality and essence, in order to avoid the greater risks of recurrent illness, fertility difficulties, or chronic pain in later life. If the Kidney essence does not adequately nourish the bones and nerves and brain during childhood and adolescent growth, poor memory and concentration can result. The adult may not have the endurance for long periods of work or the drive to pursue his full potential in life.

Aaron Duffy, an intelligent and humorous professor of comparative literature, was born to a forty-six-year-old mother and sixty-two-year-old father. His mantra of survival is "It takes me longer to do everything." Aaron is observant, insightful, articulate, and accomplished in academic and professional matters. He is very patient and kind with his students. He can display a cutting wit when in friendly company, but is guarded and usually silent in larger groups. He has a lifelong history of limited physical stamina,

---

forty-five minutes. It stops their world. They get to experience a period full of wonderful healing molecules and deep rest and balance. Instead of a state of aggravation or agitation, it is a state of wholeness and wellness. Being able to stimulate this state makes me feel like the doctor I want to be.—*John Adams, M.D.*

With acupuncture I am challenged to evaluate patients from both occidental and oriental traditions. One of the most exciting features has been seeing how acupuncture

easy weight gain, food intolerances, distance and reading vision problems, back pain, and low sex drive. He protects himself through careful diet and rest, judiciously guarding his energy output, and the regular practice of Qi Gong. By following these precautions he has been able to enjoy a fulfilling professional and family life.

Kidney essence is the source of life. It nourishes and activates all other organs. Any chronic condition, whether musculoskeletal pain, an internal organ problem, even chronic depression, will debilitate the Kidney vitality. When Kidney essence is weakened, other organs are vulnerable to expressing their disturbances. Conversely, when another organ is disturbed, its problem drains Kidney energy. The fatigue and discouragement that come with chronic pain are the clearest manifestations of this phenomenon. The more chronic the pain, the more depleted the Kidney and the greater the resulting fatigue and discouragement.

Lifestyle also influences the quality and quantity of essence. In our American culture, Kidney depletion is commonly caused by extended periods of physical and mental overwork. This lifestyle is not only expected of us, but is often eagerly sought by strong and willful people. The long hours, constant stress, irregular eating, and lack of physical exercise can take a toll on the Kidney from which it might never fully recover. If excessive sexual activity is included in the equation, the cost in essence is even higher.

In adults, an early sign of Kidney energy fatigue arises as the dark or puffy circles that appear under the eyes when someone has been working very hard or has not been sleeping well or enough. These circles can be accompanied by an increased sensitivity to cold, requiring extra clothing during the day and additional blankets at night. Such a person

---

can help prevent the onset of diseases with appropriate and timely interventions. Of course, this also requires the cooperation of patients to take care of themselves.— *Mitchell Elkiss, D.O.*

Acupuncture has given me a sense of feeling less an invalid and more empowered on my own. The psychological impact is my ability to identify a depression or a down feeling as an early symptom. I was never able to notice that before, because I had to

can feel chilly all the time and is most comfortable curled up under a blanket with a hot water bottle or heating pad. An unrelieved state of exhaustion can lead to discouragement and lack of interest in outside activities. The exhaustion can extend into the reproductive sphere as well, diminishing interest in sexual activity or impairing sexual function. The quality of quiet caution that is characteristic of the healthy Kidney-Water personality can lapse into a fearfulness that inhibits interacting with other people. Such a person might be secretly jealous or misanthropic and could be perceived as detached, cynical, and even paranoid.

Kidney deficient people characteristically prefer clothing that is dark blue or black, have a strong craving for salty food, and easily slip into speech patterns that sound groaning and complaining. They may be pallid or gray and chronically tired. The salt craving, whether it is acted on or not, is the body's innate attempt to nourish or stimulate the depleted Kidney. The quality of Kidney energy is reflected in the thickness, moistness, and color of the head hair. Poorly nourished hair is dull, thin, and brittle. Those who gray or bald before their fifth decade are probably demonstrating an inherited Kidney deficiency, unless they have acquired this state through illness, trauma, overwork, or overindulgence. We have all observed people graying suddenly during or following a period of great emotional stress.

Of course, the Kidney also supervises the filtering of blood to remove impurities and thereby maintain fluid and electrolyte balance. Kidney stones, urinary tract infections, prostate swelling and inflammation, and urination problems of dribbling and incontinence are all disharmonies of Kidney energy. Finally, Kidney nourishes the ears and the sense of hearing. The Kidney-Water type can be very sensitive to

---

deny that it was there, because before I didn't have anything but mega-antibiotics to treat me. Now I have a more refined range of symptoms to read, and thus intervention can be more timely and effective. The art of healing seems to be reemerging through medical acupuncture.—*Mary Wilson*
I think the path ahead is integrating acupuncture, cranial osteopathic work, homeopathy, and Chinese herbs to produce a new type of general medicine. It's now called

sounds and noise and music. Hearing loss, balance problems, and ringing in the ears usually reflect a disturbance in Kidney energy. This is especially the case if the hearing loss appears early in life.

Kidney vitality diminishes with age, and many of the changes associated with aging are caused by this deficiency. These can include gray hair, hearing loss, diminished sexual function, and osteoporosis. One of Kidney's most important responsibilities – the bones and joints – reflects these gradual changes. As we age, we become increasingly aware of stiffness and contractions in our bodies. The joint aches are worse in the morning and in cold weather, better after a hot shower or bath and some gentle movement, less bothersome in warm weather. Although the joint pains can be erratic and migrate from one location to another, the knees are the classical first site to demonstrate Kidney-related joint discomfort. Then the low back, the upper back, and neck become involved. The back pain typical of Kidney deficiency tends to be recurrent or chronic, and dull and aching in nature. It is commonly accompanied by deterioration in the bones of the spine when viewed on X-rays. Onset of these chronic arthritic problems earlier than the fifties or sixties suggests Kidney fatigue early in life.

Elena Verde embodies all the favorable qualities of the Water constitution. She worked for years as a professional typist and word-processor, and spent many weekends watching and counting birds with the Audubon Society. Elena is reliable and quiet, and she imposes her opinion only when she sees it is necessary for the family or group to accomplish its goal. She also embodies the signs and symptoms of the Water biopsychotype as she moves through her seventh and eighth decades. She comes in to be treated

---

complementary or alternative or integrative, but it operates from general principles that are true forever, rather than changing every five years. It is also more in keeping with the call of being a physician.—*John Adams, M.D.*
People need a different vision of health. Acupuncture can help with that vision because it is an instrument to open health and life. The sooner we can identify medical acupuncture as something that has been incorporated into conventional medicine rather

for arthritic pains in her neck, low back, thumbs, and knees. She feels chilly more easily now than in the past, gets fatigued from large family gatherings, experienced a decreased interest in sexual activity in her mid-forties, and has trouble hearing some of the birds that she used to recognize easily. Most recently she came in with a urinary tract infection that was caused by not drinking enough and voiding enough during a long bird-watching outing. Her mother was my patient for the twenty years before her death and manifested the same Kidney-Water constitution, with low back pain and hip arthritis.

Biopsychotypes Revisited

This concludes the tour of the human organism as organized from the perspective of constitutional biopsychotypes. I find the beauty of this approach to be its descriptions of the healthy qualities that make each of us unique. We are different one from the other. This is neither good nor bad; it's just the way it is.

Most conventional medical training concentrates on pathology, on what is not right with us. Physicians uninitiated in the discipline of acupuncture are trained to look only at what's wrong, at what parts have broken down, and then try their best to fix them. They are not trained to embrace the diverse presentations of balanced and healthy people before their conditions evolve into illness. For this reason alone, I think that the wisdom of acupuncture holds great value for you and for your doctor.

As you start to incorporate the model of biopsychotypes into your observations of yourself, you will be able to identify features of organs and elements that are not pathology, that are part of your healthy

---

than as something foreign or alien, the sooner we will have a stronger medicine.—
Joe DiPrisco

makeup. You might be uneasy at how many times in these last three chapters you have found features that apply to you, and wonder what kind of biopsychotype blend makes up your constitution. Or, if you have located yourself fairly squarely in one biopsychotype, you might wonder what you can do to take best advantage of your makeup, and to help prevent breakdown. I outline some common sense guidelines in the next chapters.

CHAPTER 8
GETTING TO KNOW *YOU*

By now you have certainly recognized some of yourself in each of the biopsychotypes. If you haven't yet identified which one of the three predominates in your constitutional makeup, then you probably wonder what to do next to figure yourself out. This chapter aims to help you do just that.

First, a few caveats. It would be rare for your makeup to be purely one biopsychotype, with no features or symptoms from the others. But it would be equally unusual if one biopsychotype did not outshine the other two in your personality, emotional patterns, and biological strengths and weaknesses. The challenge lies in identifying your preeminent biopsychotype and determining the relative proportion of each type in your constitution.

Understand that we all rely on the healthy function and interaction of all organs and systems to live our lives with optimal vitality and creativity. *Vision/Action* components supply the muscle and direction to propel us through life's projects and obstacles. *Nurture/Duty* influences quietly maintain our digestion and respiration, and thereby create energy that infuses the body. *Will/Spirit* qualities form the backbone of our organism and provide us with the spirit of self-expression. We need the contributions from all three divisions and all their organs to move successfully through life; they are at once independent and interdependent.

Characteristics or symptoms associated with the three types commonly emerge under different circumstances and at different moments in life. For example, Vision/Action manifests in the vitality of youthful activity and exploration; Nurture/Duty comes into focus with work, marriage, and parenting; and Will/Spirit motivates us throughout life, peaking in our full adulthood and gradually declining as we grow old. In this sense, we experience a common evolution of the qualities we share as human beings, regardless of our constitutional blend.

From a physician's perspective, the biopsychotypes divide the imbalances commonly treated by acupuncture into three main groups. Vision/Action problems usually emerge as muscular aches and pains, along with the stress and tension that accompany autonomic nervous system agitation. Nurture/Duty problems commonly emerge as "functional" digestive problems, or as digestive and respiratory problems that have dug in and are here to stay. Will/Spirit problems typically involve chronic bone related pain, such as comes from osteoarthritis and degenerative disc disease, along with the fatigue that accompanies any chronic illness. These are the three main categories we see in our acupuncture patients. Obviously, every person and every problem is unique. But these are the big groups into which we quickly sort our patients' difficulties, even before we address the details.

But What About *You*?

How can you better determine the balance of the different types at play in yourself? Do what I do with my patients. Start by taking a look at what bothers you most, be it a physical affliction or an emotional disharmony (what we call the "chief complaint" in the medical interview). You already know the things that bother you, and you have probably already identified links between the various small and large complaints and the organs, elements, and types with which they are affiliated. Now, which of these is the most important obstacle to your well-being? That's the chief complaint. Even if it's not a complaint that would take you to the doctor, that's where you should start your personal investigation.

I listen to the chief complaint, the details of its manifestation in the patient, how and when it started, and its evolution from the time that it was first noticed ("history of present illness"). As I hear each piece of information, I try to connect to it an organ, an element, or a biopsychotype. When there is a pause in the patient's explanation, I will prompt him with questions pertaining to the biopsychotype I see most clearly presenting itself in the his or her symptoms.

You can do this for yourself, whether the issue you're considering is big or small. Ask yourself questions from the three biopsychotypes to determine how strongly your features or problems are linked to one type and how powerfully that type contributes to your overall makeup. Start with the type associated with your most prominent feature or persistent symptom, even if it turns out not to be the predominant type in your constitution. Let's go through the biopsychotypes one-by-one, with explanations for the "why" of each group of questions.

Vision/Action

The balanced Vision/Action state includes many key features, most of them associated with the Wood element, but with some Fire in the background. Ask yourself what your strong points are. Do they, even in a most general way, coincide with some items on this list?

Are you:
- good at making decisions and planning things?
- usually working on a project, at home and at work?
- aware of everything that's going on around you?
- limber and well coordinated?
- energetic, confident, and usually in good spirits?
- pretty good at sports?

Do you:
- expect that whatever you set out to do will work out?
- know where everything is at your work area, even though it might look disorganized to others?
- like sports because you like the movement and discipline?
- have strong fingernails?
- have good eyesight?
- have easy digestion?

Have you:

- developed your natural visual skills in your professional or personal activities?
- done a good job organizing the apartment or house where you live?
- done a good job of arranging your work area?

It is important to consider the affiliations of the elements in each biopsychotype as you go through this inventory. The Wood element has color, flavor, and season affinities that you might encounter in yourself—strongly, slightly, or not at all. The color range for Wood includes blue, green, and turquoise. Consider the color of clothing you're drawn to, the color in paintings that attract you, the color you'd prefer to surround you in a room. If you favor sour (vinegar, pickles) or citrus (grapefruit, lemons) flavors, then you possess some Wood qualities. Wood's best, or worst, season is spring. If spring is your favorite season, but that's when your ailments get worse, then you have some Wood qualities. Finally, does a walk in the wind exhilarate you, or exhaust you and leave you irritated? These are other Wood characteristics.

Or perhaps you have more Fire qualities than Wood. The Fire color preference spans red, pink, and purple, usually strong colors. And Fire's flavor preference is bitter or burned, like roasted coffee or bitter herbs. Do you prefer summer to spring or a hot climate to a temperate climate? Then you belong more in the Fire realm of Vision/Action. Remember, however, that sometimes the answers to the element questions can be capricious and inconsistent. So don't let these preferences override other qualities you're more certain of.

Now that we've considered basic traits that lead you toward a Vision/Action classification, let's take a look at the problems to which Vision/Action types are predisposed. Answering "Yes" to some of the following questions suggests that you are experiencing a disturbance in the balanced Vision/Action state, an exaggeration from the healthy configuration to the early stages of a disorder.

Do you feel:

- that your muscles are stiff, inflamed, painful, or in spasm? Do the muscles tense up in your head, neck, or jaw?
- anxious, frustrated, or agitated more often than you would like? Must you constantly work at keeping these feelings under control?
- that if you do not get exercise you will not be able to relax?
- locked up inside yourself and too anxious to say anything?
- that your underarms perspire easily, even without doing anything to work up a sweat? Do your palms sweat easily?

Do you have worrisome, nervous, or unhealthy habits, such as:

- tapping your fingers, pacing, clicking a pen, biting your nails?
- drinking alcohol to calm yourself down?
- needing coffee (or a caffeinated drink) to get going or keep going?
- drinking coffee (or a caffeinated drink) to make headaches go away?
- craving the buzz you get from coffee, tea, or dark chocolate?

Do other people see you as:

- high-strung or nervous?
- timid, reticent to express yourself?
- hypochondriacal?

Do you have:

- outbursts of anger when you're irritated with someone, even though normally you get along well with people?
- frequent days when you are short-tempered and irritable?
- problems with your eyes?
- problems with your digestion?
- frequent headaches?
- problems with your periods?
- soft nails that split or break easily?

These symptoms derive from stagnant Liver Qi. If some of your Yes answers to these questions are fairly strong or charged with emotion, you may be experiencing a deeper or ongoing disturbance within the Vision/Action sphere. Should this be the case, it is worthwhile to continue this line of questioning. If you haven't given very strong affirmative answers to the questions so far, it's unlikely you'll find more of yourself in this final list, which includes the more bothersome symptoms of rising Liver Fire. And liver-gallbladder organ problems.

When interacting with the rest of the world, do you:

- try to avoid being noticed, because you really don't like to be seen or questioned?
- always notice what other people are doing wrong?
- remember the people who have crossed you or irritated you? For a long time?
- need to push your frustration and annoyance deep inside so no one sees it?
- have trouble making quick decisions or getting things done?
- have a hard time apologizing or forgiving?
- get angry with other drivers on the road?

In terms of physical well-being, do you:

- have trouble with your eyes or vision?
- feel tight and tense somewhere in your muscles almost all the time?
- suffer repeatedly from headaches or migraines?
- have trouble falling asleep or staying asleep?
- feel your heart pounding or beating fast?
- have difficulty digesting rich or fatty meals?
- experience fullness or pain in the liver area under the right ribcage?
- have frequent but unpredictable problems with your digestion?
- drink too much caffeine for your nerves?
- use alcohol to calm your mood, too much or too often?

Use your responses to these Vision/Action questions to gauge for yourself how much of this biopsychotype is present in your constitutional makeup. Don't worry about keeping a tally right now. If you need a numerical value for each type so you can compare them, Appendix II has a questionnaire with these Vision/Action considerations, along with those for the two other types.

To complete your analysis, mentally go through the problems that have inconvenienced you enough to still remember them or that have driven you to seek medical attention ("past medical history"). Think through your health as a child and adolescent ("childhood illnesses") and that of your immediate family ("family medical history"). Does any of this information resonate with the questions you've already answered? If Vision/Action is a big part of your makeup, you'll find helpful advice on how to get and stay balanced in Chapter 9. For now, though, read on to discover just how much Nurture/Duty and Will/Spirit you might have.

Nurture/Duty

Let's follow the same sequence of questions regarding the balanced and unbalanced states of this biopsychotype. The balanced Nurture/Duty state can be linked with either the Earth element or the Metal element or be a mixture of both. How many of your strong points appear on this list?

Are you:

- well organized and neat?
- disciplined?
- rational, good at solving practical problems?
- stable, conscientious, and responsible?
- thrifty?
- loyal?
- nurturing?
- calm?
- easygoing?

Do you:

- have a soothing or melodic voice?
- like to cook? Like to eat?
- digest your meals easily?
- enjoy the good things in life – good food, good friends, good fun?
- make sure the people with you are having a good time?
- like to greet your friends with a hug?
- feel that taking care of your family is the most important thing you can do?
- get involved in community or religious activities?
- get the job done, on time, with the details right?
- have neat handwriting?
- tend to stick to your routines and habits?
- have a tone of voice that sounds as if you know what you're talking about?

Can you:

- concentrate and stay focused on what you have to do?
- memorize a lot of information?
- express exactly what you have in mind to other people?
- remember a lot of details that people tell you about their lives?

The "Are you?" questions in this list start with Metal qualities and evolve into Earth qualities. The "Do you?" questions start with Earth and move into Metal. If Nurture/Duty forms a significant part of your makeup, you have probably noticed that you have qualities linked with both the Metal and Earth elements.

Do you like colors in the range of yellow, ochre, and earth tones? Are you drawn to sweets, or to starches and carbohydrates, and especially to milk chocolate? If so, you are identifying some of the Earth qualities of Nurture/Duty. The susceptible season for Earth is Indian summer, harvest time. Do you feel best during this time? Or are your problems aggravated during this transition from summer to autumn?

The color for Metal is white (which is the presence of all colors), and its season is autumn. Are you fond of well-seasoned or even piquant and spicy dishes? Do you prefer a spicy meal to a sweet dessert? Then you are most likely firmly in the Metal arena of Nurture/Duty. Don't forget: most of us contain mixed biopsychotypes or mixed elements within one biopsychotype. So don't worry if you like spicy meals *and* sweet desserts.

The following list describes imbalances in the full spectrum of Nurture/Duty's sphere, some Lung-Metal, some Spleen-Earth. Do you see yourself anywhere here?

Do you feel:

- driven to take care of everybody and everything?
- that you can be too introspective, self-absorbed, or brooding?
- as though you haven't felt well since you gave birth to your child?
- as if you easily slip into a black cloud or feel sad or melancholy?
- that you can be too self-critical and annoyed with yourself when things don't go as well as you would like them to?

Do you have worrisome or unhealthy habits, such as:

- smoking cigarettes, even though you know it's not good for you?
- being too much of a caretaker, getting overly involved in the lives and problems of other people?
- going overboard with the good things in life, eating and drinking too much?

Do other people see you as:

- taking a lot of their time telling them your problems?
- being too much of a perfectionist?

Do you have:

- the body type that takes on weight easily?
- intermittent digestive problems, such as belching, heartburn, bloating, cramping, or diarrhea?
- more colds than those around you?

- colds that quickly settle into your lungs or that take a long time to pass?
- recurrent outbreaks on your skin, such as acne or eczema (as a child or as an adult)?
- irregular or painful menstrual periods?
- a background of frequent bellyaches as a child?
- a background of frequent colds and flu as a child?

Several Yes answers mean that you have a strong presence of Nurture/Duty in your makeup. The suggestions in Chapter 10 will be instrumental in moving you off the "imbalances" list and back onto the "strong points" list.

The following list involves some of the more severe chronic disturbances that can plague the Nurture/Duty biopsychotype. These problems will probably already have driven you to a doctor for evaluation and treatment.

Do you have:

- a personality that frets and worries all the time, about yourself, your family, your friends, your colleagues, and the world?
- depression to the point of not being able to work effectively?
- obsessive or compulsive behavior that interferes with your daily activities and interactions with your family and friends?
- a habit of using substances for intoxication, such as alcohol or recreational drugs?
- heaviness in the chest, abdomen, or pelvis?
- chronic phlegmy respiratory problems, such as bronchitis, asthma, or emphysema?
- pain in the esophagus or stomach, such as acid reflux or stomach ulcers?
- chronic difficulty digesting your food, with bloating, discomfort, constipation, or diarrhea?
- very irregular periods, or times when your period has disappeared altogether?
- difficulty conceiving or carrying a pregnancy to term?

- uterine fibroids?
- chronic heaviness or swelling in the legs?
- hemorrhoids or varicose veins?
- prolapsed bladder, uterus, vagina, or rectum?
- diabetes or anemia?

As you consider the items on these Nurture/Duty lists, apply them also to your childhood health problems, problems you had as a younger adult, and problems that you see in members of your family. Even if you don't see them in yourself at the moment, the fact that they were once present in you or that members of your family are experiencing them should make you think that there is a strong presence of Nurture/Duty in your makeup.

Will/Spirit

The third biopsychotype – Will/Spirit – involves the dynamic interplay of Water and Fire qualities and the spheres of responsibility of the Kidney and the Heart. Do your strong points strike a chord with the qualities on this list, qualities that embody the balanced Will/Spirit state, with Water and Fire working harmoniously together?

Are you:
- reliable and directed?
- a good leader, or a good follower?
- level-headed? Adaptable?
- confident and decisive?
- willful? Intuitive?
- usually in good health?
- expansive, including others in things you are doing?

Do you:
- generally feel happy to be alive?
- catch on and learn quickly?
- often land in a leadership position?
- stay calm and quiet most of the time?
- enjoy playing sports because you like the competition?

- try not to let other people see your shortcomings?
- have strong bones and good teeth?
- play the role of life-of-the-party?
- like to wear brightly colored clothing?
- sometimes appear intense or speedy to other people?

Can you:

- work hard and keep going for a long time?
- quickly sympathize with others and understand their situation?

Some of the qualities in this list apply to most balanced people, no matter how much Will/Spirit is in their constitution. But it would be unusual for someone predominantly composed of one of the other biopsychotypes to possess the bulk of these characteristics or to resonate strongly with the Water or Fire elemental qualities. We reviewed the Fire qualities in the Vision/Action section of this chapter. Is your color preference in the red range? Do you favor roasted or bitter flavors over sweet, salty, sour, or spicy? How do you relate to summer weather? Do you like the heat, or is it too much for your body and psyche?

Or do you have strong Water qualities in your composition? Are you drawn to black or dark blue as a color to wear or drive in? How about flavors? Do you want to binge on salted nuts or potato chips, whether or not you indulge that impulse? Is winter a time that you like, because you enjoy being in the cold? Or a time that you dislike, because the cold stirs up symptoms that you don't enjoy?

The following questions probe the early stages of exaggeration from a balanced Will/Spirit state. They explore early symptoms of Kidney-Water deficiency and Heart-Fire excess.

Do you feel:

- that you don't have the energy to get everything done?
- that you are doubting yourself, lacking the confidence you once had?
- that you keep thinking things over but have trouble making up your mind?

- that your life is busy and successful, but often too stressful?
- that you can do outrageous things just because you feel like it? That you can do anything and get away with it?

Do other people see you as:

- moving and talking very quickly?
- passionate about what you're doing?
- being sexually very active?
- being arrogant or bossy, when you feel that you simply see how things can be done correctly sooner than others do?
- having a short fuse to your temper, but calming down quickly, and without grudges?
- ordering them around when you want to get things done on your timetable?
- being a good team member, but usually quiet in meetings and planning sessions?

Did you:

- start losing your hair in your twenties or thirties?
- start graying in your twenties or thirties?

Do you have:

- problems with your back, stiffness in your joints?
- intermittent pains in your chest, pounding heart, or dizzy spells?
- cold feet?
- trouble sleeping?
- frequent bad dreams?

Remember to ponder how you would have answered these questions when you were younger and how your family members would answer on your behalf. This will give you a sense of how strongly Will/Spirit qualities are represented in your constitutional makeup. The following questions explore the presence of deeper or long-term imbalances in the Will/Spirit sphere. These symptoms are commonly accompanied by an ongoing sense of fatigue and a lack of motivation to push very hard.

Have you:

- gone through a prolonged period of severe illness or malnutrition in your life?
- gone through prolonged periods of working too hard and exhausting yourself?
- had many ear, throat, or respiratory infections as a child?

Are you:

- more cautious or fearful than others around you?
- becoming more sensitive to noise?
- going through or recovering from a severe or prolonged illness?

In terms of physical well-being, do you:

- have dark circles or puffiness under your eyes?
- often feel chilly inside your body?
- have little interest in sexual activity?
- suffer regularly from insomnia?
- have trouble with your hearing?
- sometimes lose your balance?
- have chronic neck or back pain, with or without radiation to arms or legs?
- have degenerative or osteoarthritic changes in your spine or joints?
- have any urinary tract symptoms, such as kidney stones, frequent bladder infections, prostate problems, difficulty with urination?
- have coronary artery or cardiac disease?

If, having read through Chapters 5, 6, and 7, and the question lists in this chapter, you are still not clear about the balance of the biopsychotypes in your makeup, score the questionnaire in Appendix II to arrive at a numerical weight for each type. Use these proportions to guide your exploration of the measures you can take to stabilize the irregularities in your health. In reading the next three chapters, I suggest you start with the chapter dealing with the type that you perceive as predominant in yourself. And then read the chapter on the next strongest type, finishing with the chapter least present in you.

CHAPTER 9
LESSONS FROM VISION/ACTION

Exaggerations in the Vision/Action terrain drive people to seek professional attention outside conventional medical services for two main reasons. First, the symptoms, while not life-threatening, become chronic and interfere with quality of life and effectiveness at work. Second, conventional medical therapies offer little that directly affects these conditions without unpleasant or limiting additional effects. This is especially true of the anxiety-driven manifestations and muscular disturbances common in Vision/Action. Here are some basic steps you can take to deal with a disturbance in this biopsychotype.

Know Yourself

Understanding where you fit along the Vision/Action balance-to-disturbance spectrum allows you to plan your personal and professional activities to accommodate your individual strengths and shortcomings. Simply being aware that your confidence and drive, your organizational skills, and your potential for irritability or timidity are part of your constitutional makeup, should encourage you to work with your strengths while accommodating and overcoming your weaknesses. Understanding your characteristics and disturbances may help you integrate healthy changes into your personality and your physical condition. For example, seeing how you affect those around you should lead you to gain greater control over bothersome impulsive behavior patterns. Or, recognizing that you feel most lucid, energized, and productive when you have exercised, should lead you to include regular daily physical exercise into your work and home schedule.

If you have trouble interpreting signals from your friends or work colleagues about habits and personality qualities that they consider less than ideal, or if your impatience or anxiety constantly interferes with your interactions with these people, you can gain insight about yourself by *keeping a journal*. A journal does not have to be an elaborate or time-consuming project. When you feel out of sorts or wonder why people are reacting to you in a way that unsettles you, create a dialogue with yourself in the privacy of your journal. Try to identify the feelings or difficulties you experience and describe them in writing. Describe the situation as a conversation where you are the other person. Ponder the obstacles, think about creative ways to surmount them, and write them down. You can make this an ongoing process to clarify your internal emotional and personality issues, or you can return to the journal whenever your unsettled thoughts take you there. The act of putting words to your emotions stimulates a dialogue with your subconscious that continues even when you are not writing or thinking about writing.

The issues that you, as a Vision/Action type, are likely to face in your emotional life and your journal are the psychological consequences of stagnant Liver Qi. Challenge yourself to overcome frustration and irritability with flexibility and grace, and to overcome anger and grudge-holding with patience and forgiveness. Address your timidity with your innate courage, and the confidence derived from that courage will convert your vision and insight into plans and action. Develop an arms-length distance from your emotional impulses so you can evaluate their impact before you speak or act. Keep up your internal conversation with your journal. Your subconscious can often provide suggestions and solutions that emerge as you continue your writing. Follow them. Keep the Qi moving.

Relax, Exercise
Exercise, Relax

A relaxed psychological and physical state is essential for Vision/Action people to function effectively at home and at work. The agitation triggered by ambition and activity easily creates an emotional milieu of frustration, anxiety, impatience, and irritability. These unpleasant and unproductive emotions can in large measure be countered through relaxation and exercise. If you live at the active end of the Vision/Action spectrum, vigorous physical exercise is indispensable. You have probably already identified your favorite and most effective sports or workouts, whether they be basketball, racquetball, tennis, running, biking, swimming, Judo, aerobics, stair-climbing, or ski machine. Whatever it is, aim to *do some physical activity regularly*, at least three times a week; even better, shoot for five times. Even exercise as gentle as walking can provide the necessary repose.

If you live at the quiet end of the spectrum, you may prefer relaxation techniques, such as meditation, biofeedback, or self-hypnosis, as tools to contact a calm center within the turmoil of constant ideas and activity. Yoga breathing and postures provide one path to the calm center, and they have the added value of stretching joints and muscles. Qi-moving martial arts, such as Tai Chi Chuan and Qi Gong, are especially valuable if you have tight or stiff muscles. For all Vision/Action types, opportunities for movement must be worked into the daily routine. It is critical that you maintain a balance of activity and rest, each day, at work and at home. Go for a walk after lunch or during your morning and afternoon breaks. Join a gym close to work. Exchange massages with family and friends to reduce the muscle tension and inflammation that come with this constitutional territory. If you're on your own, you can benefit from electric massaging equipment now widely available. However you can, keep the Qi and blood flowing.

Eat Well

In acupuncture and Chinese traditional medicine, the fundamental concept in treatment is to provide a stimulus that is equal but opposite to the problem being addressed. We design needle patterns to move stagnant Liver Qi and to disperse the Fire of a headache. We prescribe herbal formulas to address the same disharmonies of stagnant Qi and excess Fire. We make dietary recommendations to provide nourishment that balances internal irregularities. Chinese dietary guidelines give great importance to the temperature of the food and drink you consume, and even greater attention to the temperature and internal moisture a food produces as you digest it. Foods can be cold- or cool-producing, warmth- or heat-producing, damp-producing, or neutral, depending on the effect they have on internal temperature and moisture when digested. Foods chosen according to these attributes help restore a disturbed condition to a state of balance.

If you find yourself expending energy and attention keeping anxiety and irritability in check, limit your intake of foods that cause Liver stagnation and Liver Fire. Cut back on rich or fatty meals, high-fat foods (cookies, pastries, crackers, products containing margarine or vegetable shortening), deep-fried foods (including fried fast food, French fries, doughnuts), whole milk and dairy products (such as butter, cream, cheese, ice cream), and hot and spicy sauces and curries. You might crave spicy foods, because they stimulate Qi and temporarily resolve the feeling of Liver stagnation, but too much hot spice risks fanning a stagnant Liver condition into a raging Liver Fire.

If you must eat some fried food, be sure to include sour flavors with it. Sour and acid flavors reduce the Liver excesses and help to balance the effects of rich food. Sour foods include lemons, limes, sour apples, vinegar, pickles, olives, sauerkraut, leeks, tomatoes, and green mangoes. Liver stagnation can also be overcome by eating fresh greens and sprouts and by using pungent cooking herbs, such as basil, fennel, marjoram, rosemary, caraway, bay leaf, cardamom, cumin, and ginger.

Eat your biggest meal in the middle of the day or in the afternoon, and avoid late night meals. Avoid eating quickly or overeating; both create stagnation in the stomach and intestines. Overeating heavy or hard-to-digest food like nuts, nut butters, and meat also retards digestion and can weakens Liver Qi. Likewise, skipping meals or eating on the run adds to autonomic nervous system stress and overburdens the Liver. Sit down and relax during your meals. Moderation keeps the Qi flowing.

As a Vision/Action person, one of your greatest lifestyle issues will be your consumption of caffeine stimulants and alcohol. You probably like the energy kick-start of caffeine in the morning and possibly would like more than a few boosters during the day. Caffeine can help you focus and keep your day moving. But caffeine also taxes the Liver and autonomic nervous system, and, when used to excess, can generate all the symptoms of Liver Qi stagnation and Liver Fire. Recognize what "excess" is for your own well-being, and stay well below that level.

Living as intensely as you like to, you probably find alcohol useful as a rapid mood-changer when your workday is over. You might also find that when a little feels good, more feels even better. Define a safe and reasonable limit to your alcohol consumption. Measure your drinks; stay within your limits. Excess alcohol impedes the Liver Qi; moderation keeps the Qi flowing.

In general, most people remain healthy when they eat primarily warming foods cooked fresh and eaten warm; lots of fresh vegetables eaten warm; grains and fiber; a variety of animal proteins; moderate amounts of nuts, seeds, and fruits; and not much concentrated sweet or fat. Try preparing your meals with whole foods – that is, food that is fresh, not processed, without preservatives or refined sugars. It is especially important to eat warmer foods during winter months or in cold climates and cooler foods during the summer. In dietary therapy, it is important not to take recommendations to such an extreme that the demands of the new diet will further tax or deplete the digestive process. For example, although cool- and cold-producing foods are good for a hot summer or a hot internal disease, eating too many cooling and cold foods may slow down the digestive process and diminish the useful Qi derived from the diet.

Seek Treatment

If your muscle tension, headache, anxiety, or irritability do not resolve with introspection, relaxation, exercise, or dietary activities, consider seeking professional intervention to help you in your repair process. There are several useful options in the conventional and complementary disciplines.

Acupuncture relieves the acute muscle pains and emotional strains brought on by the stresses and tensions of our daily lives. Acute muscle spasm can often be relieved with one or two treatments. If your constitution is primarily Vision/Action, however, your acute problems typically occur superimposed on chronic anxiety states and pain from tight muscles. If this is your situation, incorporating regular acupuncture sessions into your health maintenance can keep pains and spasms at bay. Monthly treatments create a useful fundamental rhythm, and additional visits can be requested when you slip out of balance (which will happen when you have a new deadline at work or a difficult personal situation).

Acupuncture for musculoskeletal pain and recurrent headaches includes needle stimulation, often with electricity, and probably other traditional techniques that help move stagnant blood and Qi in the muscles, such as spoon scraping. *Spoon scraping* involves deeply massaging the tight muscles with the smooth edge of a Chinese soup spoon, pressing firmly enough to force the blood to move through the muscles. This technique might seem strange, but for those who need it the deep massage feels as if it's warming and relaxing the muscles, like it's a "good hurt." It is a treatment that is best done regularly, even weekly, to keep the tight zones relaxed and mobile. I recommend training someone in your family to be the official weekly scraper.

If your muscular problems persist despite acupuncture therapy, look for a practitioner in the *manual medicine* arts whose work complements the acupuncture. Your physician acupuncturist will probably be able to refer you to a reliable provider. This might be a physician practicing osteopathic manipulative therapy whose techniques can influence bone alignment, joint function, and muscle holding patterns better than acupuncture alone. Some registered physical therapists have additional qualifications in osteopathic techniques. A physical therapist or a massage therapist trained in myotherapy can add deep tissue massage to the equation and help break up the deep connective tissue and muscle holding patterns. You may pursue any of these manual medicine approaches in conjunction with the acupuncture treatments until the pain patterns have been resolved or at least controlled. Of course, during and after the period of acupuncture and manual medicine treatments, you still need to incorporate the stretching and strengthening exercises recommended for your musculoskeletal problem.

Acupuncture also effectively reduces the anxiety, irritability, and agitation that accompany muscle pains. One common approach is to treat the agitated mental state during the first part of the session, then treat the musculoskeletal problem during the second part. This way, both psychology and body are treated with appropriate needle patterns at the same office visit. While acupuncture can be very effective in creating a psychological "vacation" from the experience of anxiety and inner tension, if the external and internal drivers of the anxiety are not modified, the psychological benefits of the treatment will wear off quickly.

If the emotional symptoms of stagnant Liver Qi have become chronically inconvenient or inappropriate, adding *Chinese herbal formulations* to your treatment program can be very effective. Several U.S.-based companies produce classical Chinese herbal formulas in safe, effective, and easy-to-use preparations of pills, tinctures, and powders. Several herbal combinations are tailor-made to move Liver Qi, move blood and Qi through the channels, or calm Liver Fire. Herbal prescribing is not a standard component of medical acupuncture training for physicians, although physicians are increasingly seeking this training. Many licensed acupuncturists qualified in traditional Chinese acupuncture are also qualified to prescribe Chinese herbs.

Herbs can address both emotional and physical symptoms of the Vision/Action biopsychotype. They treat the Liver energy problems without contaminating the body's metabolism or nervous system. Typically, for herbal preparations to prove effective in improving your symptoms, they require an extended period of use to create an enduring change. The herbs work hand-in-hand with acupuncture, since they add a daily therapy aimed at changing the same problems being addressed with the periodic acupuncture treatments.

Constitutional homeopathy is another therapeutic approach to consider for the psychoemotional component of Vision/Action symptoms, especially if your anxiety and irritability continue to impair your comfortable interaction with friends and colleagues. Homeopathic remedies address chronic disturbances on an energetic level that is subtler than the energy impact of acupuncture. A well-prescribed homeopathic remedy may modify the psychological dynamics to achieve a level of greater comfort and function. Symptomatic acupuncture for muscular pain may be continued while taking a homeopathic remedy.

More deep-seated and troublesome psychoemotional dynamics that keep you frustrated or anxious can, of course, be mollified with *anti-anxiety and anti-depressant medication.* Please consider these drugs only after you have genuinely attempted to help yourself with the approaches already discussed. Don't rush to use them until you have tested the results of the other treatments for your problem. On the other hand, don't be reluctant to use them if your problems are simply not responding to other approaches. These medications can be a valuable part of the symptomatic treatment for Vision/Action challenges; however, they can also bring unwanted physiological and psychological effects. Using appropriate anti-anxiety or anti-depressant drugs does not interfere with the acupuncture response. In fact, they can facilitate a longer-lasting change in difficult muscle pain patterns by modifying the neurological response to pain.

Because the Vision/Action terrain serves as the sensitive interface between psyche and soma, common sense health care dictates that we reduce the symptoms of stagnation by maintaining balance in our daily activities. It is critical that we understand how we function and under what circumstances our disturbances appear. More importantly, we need to know what we can do to return the early disturbances to normal or at least keep them in check. Maintain a reasonable pace and set limits that reduce the symptoms of stress and tension overload.

Relaxation, exercise, a good diet, acupuncture, manual therapy, herbs, homeopathy, pharmaceuticals…find what works for you to keep the Qi moving and to keep your Vision/Action self in balance.

CHAPTER 10
LESSONS FROM NURTURE/DUTY

Nurture/Duty people typically seek acupuncture or complementary medical attention because they are tired of being repeatedly or chronically plagued with digestive or respiratory disorders. They are also reluctant to accept lifelong prescriptions of antibiotics, corticosteroids, antacids, antispasmodics, achlorhydrics, and antidepressants to pacify their problems. Conventional medical management offers little hope of reversal or cure once an organ-based diagnosis has been established. Even before looking for outside help, you can do a lot for yourself by recognizing early symptoms and managing them with self-understanding, diet, and exercise. The first step is to focus some of your innate caring and responsibility on yourself. The second step is to identify those foods that help maintain a happy Spleen and healthy digestion.

Know Yourself

Begin by identifying where your personality fits along the Earth-to-Metal continuum of Nurture/Duty features and, by careful reflection, ascertaining which of your qualities are strengths and which might better be viewed as indulgences or shortcomings. The compassion and abundance of Earth can slip into over-nurturing or self-absorption. Do you spend a lot of your time in the role of understanding confidante, or find yourself solving other people's problems, being everything to everyone? Do you have trouble saying "No" to commitments that inevitably become more complicated and stickier than you have time for? Do you tend to brood, or wallow in self-pity?

The meticulousness and perfectionism of Metal can become self-critical and judgmental. Do you expect the impossible from yourself and then dwell only on your shortcomings? Have you been accused of trying to control everyone and everything around you? Do you fall easily into a melancholy mood? And then impose this mood on others? Have you noticed that during the past year or so you have had more times of dissatisfaction than satisfaction with your personality and your life? And have you had more respiratory infections or digestive upsets during this time?

If you answer "Yes" to more than a few of these questions, and especially if you feel isolated and unable to analyze or break the habit, *working with a journal* may give you the insight you need. Putting words to your feelings and concerns about yourself and others can clarify which issues matter to you and which you can set aside. A relationship with your journal can reveal aspects of yourself as others see you, and thereby help you modify your style of interacting with the people who are important to you. If your impulse to rescue all your friends is confined to your journal, you will recover a wealth of reserve energy, balance, and time. If, in the course of your journal writing, you recognize that the world will go on even if you're not involved in every detail, those around you will be able to relax along with you.

As a Nurture/Duty type, you will need to address – whether by self-evaluation or journal-writing – issues of involvement, control, organization, mood, and indulgence. Call on your courage to keep your empathy in balance and on your confidence to soften your self-absorption. Figure out how to extricate yourself from sticky situations without severing your connection with family, friends, and colleagues. Aim at excellence, but embrace forgiveness and goodwill when you or others fall short of the mark. Use good humor to overcome melancholy; offer a smile rather than a snarl when you're feeling blue, and you'll get back warmth and a smile in return. Most important and most difficult of all, maintain a balance between order and the pursuit of pleasure. Nourish your Qi, and keep it flowing.

Eat Well

If you are an Earth Nurture/Duty person, you already know that you love to eat and spend a lot of time thinking about, preparing, and eating good food. You also know that you can easily skid into overeating and have trouble maintaining a healthy weight. Earth people have big appetites for food and pleasure, and especially for sweets. Your constitutional tendency to gravitate toward comfort, abundance, and involvement risks fostering an atmosphere of overindulgence and lassitude. These characteristics create a recipe for life-long conflict between enjoyment and moderation.

Remember, most people remain healthy if they eat primarily warming foods cooked fresh and eaten warm; lots of fresh vegetables eaten warm; grains and fiber; a variety of animal protein; moderate amounts of nuts, seeds, and fruits; and few concentrated sweets or fats. The Spleen, which supervises the digestive process, is especially vulnerable to cold-producing and damp-producing foods. These foods create sluggishness and stagnation in the Stomach and prevent the Spleen from extracting all the nutrition from the food. To complicate life for Earth types trying to lose weight, popular dieting practices insist that eating copious quantities of raw vegetables and uncooked fruit is unquestionably the most effective regime. On the contrary, this is the worst diet possible for Nurture/Duty people. The Spleen and Stomach cannot process so much cold and damp food. Such a diet results in a state of digestive sluggishness and tissue dampness, and little nourishing energy is derived from the process.

For Nurture/Duty types, the American "refrigerator syndrome" is the most damaging factor in our culture's eating habits. We eat straight out of the refrigerator, add ice to everything we drink, and make uncooked or processed foods the mainstay of our diet. Iced foods and drinks (ice cream, frozen yogurt, iced water and tea, chilled milk and juices, smoothies, sodas) and unheated foods (raw salads, raw vegetables, and uncooked fruits) cannot reach the temperature inside the stomach necessary for thorough digestion before they pass into the intestines. This can result in internal cold and dampness and can lead to chronic digestive problems. Energetically cool and cold foods include lettuce, celery, cucumbers, watermelon, spinach, and tomatoes. Tofu, the vegetarian's champion substitute for animal protein, is notoriously cold-producing as well. Dairy, wheat, and sugar (milk, butter, cream, cheese, yogurt, white bread, pasta, bagels, muffins, cookies, pies, candy) and citrus fruits and juices are also damp-producing foods. Earth-Spleen types are better off minimizing this entire menu of cold, damp options.

The consequences of ingesting cold- and damp-producing foods extend beyond digestive disturbances. If the Spleen cannot clear the damp from the food in the Stomach and send nourishing energy to the Lung, the Lung becomes damp as well. Phlegm in the Lung creates thick sputum, chronic cough, and a sense of fullness in the chest. The mucus condition is worsened by dairy products, cold raw food, fried food, and alcohol.

It's not just what you eat that can tax the Spleen and damage digestion. It's also how you eat. Moderation is the most important goal for an Earth person, since it is so easy to consume too much food, too many sauces, too much sugar, milk, alcohol, and chocolate. Sit down and relax during your meal. Set aside those work worries and end the family arguments. Don't eat fast, or late at night. Eat your food warm or at least at room temperature. Take smaller servings and avoid second helpings. Chew your food well. Avoid drinking too many liquids at meals. (Drinking lots of warm fluids is very important to digestive health, but these should be taken between meals, not while the food is digesting.) Rest for a few minutes to allow what you've eaten to register before asking for additional food. You'll often find that you don't need more to feel satisfied.

Sweet foods generally have a warming effect when eaten in moderation, but not food sweetened with refined sugar. The natural sweetness of grains, fruits, and vegetables is stimulating to the Spleen and Stomach. Sweet foods include whole grains, peas, beans, lentils, fruits, beets, carrots, onions, squash, parsnips, potatoes, and sweet potatoes. These foods, eaten warm, will stabilize blood sugar levels and reduce cravings for concentrated sugars. But beware: excess sweets, even from all-natural foods, can weaken Spleen Qi and lead to weight gain and respiratory problems.

Warming foods and warm spices help the Spleen complete its digestive process; they are especially helpful when Spleen energy is deficient. Soups and stews with potatoes, leeks, onions, garlic, rice, and oats are recommended, with lean chicken, turkey, lamb, or beef. Warming spices include mustard, black pepper, cumin, turmeric, coriander, cardamom, ginger, cinnamon, nutmeg, cloves, and orange peel. Warmth and moderation maximize the Spleen Qi, sustaining the harmony you need for optimal health.

All these recommendations are especially important for anyone who already has digestive symptoms or the beginnings of Spleen deficiency. They are also important for the functions of the Lung, which falter in a damp and phlegm-filled environment. Lung-Metal types can have a metabolism that is contrary to that of their Spleen-Earth friends, even if their psychological and other physical characteristics overlap. They often have strong digestion and hypermetabolism that allow them to eat as often and as much as they want, yet not gain weight. Their Spleen-Earth relations find this an unfair genetic trick. On the other hand, the Lung-Metal types tend to be quite vulnerable to food sensitivities and allergies and are likelier than Spleen-Earth types to develop hives, eczema, sinus and bronchial congestion, wheezing, bloating, cramps, and diarrhea. Common allergy-producing foods are dairy products, foods with wheat flour, nuts, eggs, shellfish, chocolate, sugar, and citrus.

Relax, Exercise

As a fairly balanced Nurture/Duty person, you probably have a sturdy constitution but you lack the discipline to engage in regular exercise. Unlike Vision/Action people, who need a lot of physical activity to keep themselves in balance, you need exercise to remind you that you have a physical body and that this body needs attention. Regular movement helps your Spleen to develop Qi and your Lungs to propel it. You might need a kick to get going, but once you're involved in some form of regular exercise, you'll experience its psychological and physical benefits with clearer thoughts, uplifted spirits, and a body that feels lighter and more flexible.

So get off your duff and get outside. Begin with gentle walking and work up to a pace and distance that you can realistically maintain for at least thirty minutes three to five times a week. If walking isn't your thing, learn a discipline that combines breathing and stretching, such as yoga or the gentle movements of Tai Chi Chuan. Or take up ballroom dancing and do it at home as well as in class. As your strength and stamina increase, experiment with more vigorous activities, such as bicycling, swimming, hiking, and light aerobic classes. The energy and relaxation you gain from exercise will improve your digestion and keep the Spleen Qi and Lung Qi moving.

Seek Treatment

If your digestive or respiratory disturbances have been around long enough to dig in and become chronic, you may need more powerful interventions to reverse the imbalance. Persist in addressing the psychological underpinnings of the problem, stick to the diet and exercise guidelines, and decide where to turn for professional help. Here are some possibilities.

Acupuncture can slow down, reverse, or cure many of the early functional imbalances in the Nurture/Duty sphere. I emphasize *early*, because once a disturbance reaches the state of an official diagnosis, the digestive organs have already sustained some damage. The more severe the damage, the less likely it is that acupuncture alone will restore you to a normal state. Acupuncture is a good first step, though, to test the responsiveness of your problem. An acute respiratory or digestive problem, such as a recent bronchitis or gastritis, often responds promptly to several acupuncture sessions. A longer-standing problem, however, usually requires a longer series of treatments before its enduring changes can be evaluated. Commit to a dozen visits with your physician acupuncturist.

If four to six acupuncture treatments have not brought convincing changes in your condition, it may be time to add **Chinese herbal tonics** to your treatment. Excellent classical formulas from American manufacturers can relieve deficient Spleen Qi, stagnation and dampness in the digestive tract, phlegm in the chest, and weak Lung Qi. When including Chinese herbs for Spleen-Stomach problems, the first step is to restore the Spleen's transforming function sufficiently for the herbs to be digested and assimilated. Only then can the other benefits from herbal formulas emerge.

Chronic digestive problems require a long course of herbal therapy and possibly ongoing administration of a basic formula, depending on the extent and stability of the response. Likewise, when extensive chronic respiratory problems have come under control, a low-dose maintenance schedule is often required to sustain the improvements, with additional dosages or formulas brought in during vulnerable seasons or at the first hint of imbalance. Acupuncture and Chinese herbal prescriptions work hand-in-hand for chronic digestive and respiratory problems. The herbs create a sturdier response to the acupuncture energetic therapy and sustain the response with fewer acupuncture treatments, compared with acupuncture alone.

For symptoms of food sensitivities and allergies, try ***nutritional counseling*** with a physician or acupuncturist trained in nutrition, with a naturopathic practitioner, or with a holistic nutritionist. In addition to dietary counseling, nutritional therapy will include a supervised elimination and provocation diet that tests your responses to the various common food culprits, as well as nutritional supplementation to fortify your digestive and immune systems.

Osteopathic manipulative therapy can also complement the acupuncture management of chronic digestive problems. The viscera generating the inflammation or malfunction create a reflex response in the muscles of the back through which the nerves travel. You might not notice this muscle tension, or you might experience a simple muscle ache or stiffness in your lower thoracic and upper lumbar region. Or severe cramping pain may send you to bed. Osteopathic manipulation of the back muscles, and of the stomach and intestines through pressure on the abdominal muscles, can bring substantial relief for the muscular component of the problem and reduce the visceral discomfort. Musculoskeletal acupuncture techniques work nicely in conjunction with this approach.

Digestion, assimilation, and energy production form the core of our daily physical vitality. The wisdom of acupuncture can help you enhance your digestive and respiratory functions on the way to achieving optimal health. Remember, moderation in behavior, diet, and exercise keeps the Qi happy and flowing to nourish all the organs and tissues of the body.

CHAPTER 11
LESSONS FROM WILL/SPIRIT

If your biopsychotype includes a good measure of Will/Spirit, you will by now have developed a sense of how much of you is Water and how much is Fire. Understanding your constitutional components is the first step to using the wisdom of acupuncture to help you with your health and happiness. In addition to evaluating some of your personality and lifestyle habits, you'll need to consider what exercise best suits your needs and what diet most helps or hinders your health.

Know Yourself

The impulses of Will and Spirit demand attention. Your friends and colleagues probably find that these impulses in you are difficult to ignore or even painful to tolerate. Now is a good time to evaluate your effect on the other people in your life. Writing down your thoughts in a journal won't suffice. Rather, you need to observe, rehearse, and change your approach. Use your powers of perception to evaluate the responses you evoke in other people. Identify patterns of your behavior that put people off, or (if they are your subordinates) that make them mince their words. If someone close to you suggests how your interaction might be softened, don't brush it off. Listen to it. Take it in. Think about it. And try a different style next time you're with that person or in that situation.

Achieving an understanding of your impact on other people is the greatest challenge – and the most fertile ground for change – in your Will/Spirit personality. The competence, insight, creativity, enthusiasm, and authority that have brought you this far are your greatest assets. But they are also qualities that can impair your personal comfort or the comfort of those around you, and impede productive relationships when you come across as arrogant, imperious, or unsettlingly intense. Temper some of your arrogance with modesty, your imperiousness with humility, and your intensity with warmth and patience. You still have enough essence and spirit to achieve your most important goals. If you are on the excess and Fiery side of the Will/Spirit spectrum, pause to consider the likely response to what you are about to say or do. Gain some distance from your impulses and use common sense to decide if they are really worth following. Delaying your reaction is especially helpful when dealing with the passion of anger or sexual opportunity. Your Qi will move, but try to keep it in balance.

If you are on the depleted, Water side of the Will/Spirit continuum, consider creating a journal relationship to explore your sensitivities and vulnerabilities. Through *writing a journal* you can restore the stability that your depleted state has disrupted, and recover the strength to move beyond any fear that keeps you from pursuing your goals. Allow the music of the classical and romantic masters (Beethoven, Mozart, Wagner, Tchaikovsky) to bolster your inspiration and courage. If chronic pain and the fatigue from the constant discomfort of your activities dampen your spirit and deplete your essence, you risk indifference or despair. If you are forced to live with chronic pain, despite all the efforts you and others have made, refuse to allow your limitations to make you withdraw from people and activities. Tap into your inner core of Will and Spirit; stay in touch with the activities you enjoy and the people you like to be with. Accept the limitations that pain imposes on you, but practice graciousness and good will in your interactions with the people in your life. Keep your essence warm and your spirit moving.

Relax, Exercise

Burning your candle at both ends will inevitably deplete your essence and diminish your spirit. Will/Spirit people need to take time out for mental and physical relaxation. Be sure to get enough sleep. Learn breathing exercises or meditation to calm your spirit. Develop a posture that enables you to sit, stand, and walk without endangering your vulnerable back. At a minimum, keep limber with stretching, yoga, or one of the gentle martial arts, such as Tai Chi Chuan. Find an activity that you enjoy and that matches your needs, something to keep your Qi moving. Walking is always a safe, basic exercise. This can evolve to fast walking, running, or biking. If you like friendly competitive sports try volleyball or basketball. If you need to win and your back can handle it, take up racquetball, tennis, or golf. If your back tends to act up, try competitive swimming.

For both Fire and Water conditions, dancing and singing are great equalizing activities. Fire types dance to defuse pent-up energy and sing to voice their passion. Water types dance to get their Qi moving and sing to escape from their self-imposed isolation. Dancing and singing bring you into contact with others and create bonds of companionship.

If you are on the Fire end of the Will/Spirit biopsychotype, your innate creativity and drive put you at risk of depletion from willful overwork. When you are deeply engaged in activity, you can easily overlook the importance of maintaining an even pace and taking time for rest and recovery. The only position on your throttle is full speed ahead. While the exhilaration of accomplishment is personally and professionally fulfilling, the energy cost can be crippling. Learn your limits and work within them. Adequate rest can keep your spirit lively.

If you are on the Water end of the biopsychotype, you risk the consequences of depleted Kidney energy and essence. Be especially conscientious as to how you use your energy, how you exercise and rest, how you eat. If you constantly feel chilly, move into a house that is well insulated and can be kept heated, or move to a warmer climate. Avoid air conditioned buildings and automobiles and protect yourself from drafts. Practice martial arts, such as Qi Gong, that help develop and move energy in your body. Do not indulge in sexual activity more frequently than your body can recover from. Preserve your essence and keep the Qi flowing.

Eat Well

Follow the Chinese dietary guidelines for Fire and Water conditions: add cooling foods to the basic diet for Fire, and add warming foods for Water. Remember, most people remain healthy if they eat primarily warming foods cooked fresh and eaten warm; lots of fresh vegetables eaten warm; grains and fiber; a variety of animal protein;

moderate amounts of nuts, seeds, and fruits; and few concentrated sweets or fats. Also, remember not to take the recommendations of cooling or warming foods to extremes; otherwise, your diet will further tax or deplete the digestive process. Too many cold-producing foods will slow down digestion, even in a hot Fire person, and too many heat-producing foods will create internal heat symptoms, even in a cold Water person. Aim for moderation when making adjustments to the basic healthy diet of whole foods.

If your Fire features make you feel overheated, and especially if summer heat aggravates your condition, add cooling foods like raw vegetables (especially cucumbers, celery, and tomatoes), salads, uncooked fruits (especially melons), fruit and vegetable juices, yogurt, and tofu to your meals. Bitter vegetables (such as endive, kale, chard, and spinach) are considered cooling as well. Even extremes of internal heat do not, however, justify a habit of eating straight out of the refrigerator or adding ice to all your drinks. Stay away from greasy foods such as hamburgers and fries, which produce heat, and cut down on red meat, eggs, and dairy products. Avoid refined sugar, pepper, chilies, garlic, ginger, coffee, and alcohol – any of these can aggravate a heat condition. Finally, remember to drink plenty of water between meals, at room temperature or warm.

Dealing with a cold internal state does not require pursuing a diet opposite to that recommended for the hot state. Most important for the dietary support of Kidney energy is to provide the Stomach and Spleen with nutrients they can thoroughly digest and from which they can extract energy. Eat soups and stews and cooked vegetables. Add more meat and animal protein (red meat, organ meat, chicken, fish, eggs), which nourish the Kidney, and use nuts, seeds, and warming spices (such as garlic, black pepper, cinnamon, cloves, anise, and ginger) to warm the Stomach. Oatmeal and rice also add warmth. Avoid damp- and cold-producing foods such as raw vegetables, salads, and fruits, which can further chill the body. Steam or wok-fry your vegetables to make them easier to digest. A little salt is okay, but more than a taste is not good for Water types, even if you are craving it. Avoid potato chips, pretzels, ham, bacon, sausage, and canned or processed foods. And, once again, avoid refined sugar, caffeine stimulants, and especially chocolate. Like your Fire counterpart, drink plenty of water between meals.

Seek Treatment

More people come to *acupuncture* for back pain than for any other musculoskeletal, functional, or organic disorder. Most of these people inhabit Will/Spirit bodies and personalities, although back pain from injuries or the arthritic deterioration of age afflicts other biopsychotypes as well. Acupuncture is well-suited to serve as the initial approach to pain in the upper back and neck, or in the lower back. This therapy adapts well to the needs of the patient, and its effects can be enhanced by adding electrical and thermal stimulation to the needles. Patients with Kidney energy deficiency especially welcome the heat, which we provide by passing a smoldering cigar of rolled, dried mugwort (called "moxa") near the needles and over the painful region. Acupuncture may be the only therapy needed to relieve acute back pain. Maintenance acupuncture visits will likely be required in chronic pain cases.

Acupuncture can also calm agitated Fire states in the Will/Spirit individual. The Fire symptoms of agitation, insomnia, and quick anger occur because the patient has lost the balance between Water and Fire. In such cases, the Fire and spirit are easily calmed with acupuncture needle patterns, though Kidney points must be stimulated to prevent a rapid relapse to the disturbed state.

Musculoskeletal pain problems that do not show improvement within a half-dozen acupuncture sessions should be evaluated by other disciplines that complement acupuncture. *Physical therapy* techniques, for example, can significantly enhance the acupuncture treatments. Physical therapists can provide movement therapy and workplace training, both of which are indispensable to prevent a recurrence of back pain.

Of course, *osteopathic manipulative therapy* and deep tissue myotherapy are also superb complements to the acupuncture treatments. Difficult musculoskeletal pain problems can benefit from the intervention of *pain management specialists* who are qualified to perform pain-relieving procedures such as nerve blocks, epidural infiltrations, and dorsal column stimulation. These specialists are also qualified to manage the medication requirements of complex cases. Physicians with added qualifications in musculoskeletal pain management usually practice in the disciplines of anesthesiology or physical medicine (physiatry).

Chinese herbal formulas can benefit Will/Spirit problems in two ways. First, there are excellent Kidney tonics that can enhance the vitality necessary to repair and move forward from a chronic pain problem. In fact, some Chinese medicine practitioners encourage anyone over fifty years old to take herbal Kidney tonics on a regular basis, whether or not they have symptoms. Second, there are very effective formulas to calm excess Fire and ease the spirit for those dealing with the inconveniences of being overcharged and hotheaded.

Constitutional homeopathic remedies can modify emotional disturbances that prevent an agitated Fire person from contacting a calm emotional center. In deep-seated problems, psychopharmaceutical products can be used to calm the agitation of excess Fire or ameliorate the depressive component in a Kidney-depleted patient with chronic pain.

Back pain and agitated states are common problems in the Will/ Spirit population. By understanding the underlying energetic dynamics in this biopsychotype and acting on the acupuncture lessons of this chapter, you can create a more comfortable physical and psychological life for yourself. Remember, moderation keeps the Qi flowing happily.

This is the final chapter dealing with the characteristics of biopsychotypes and how to take advantage of understanding your fundamental composition. In the next three chapters I change direction, beginning with an overview of what acupuncture can best treat. This material should help you sort out acupuncture's potential value in your health issues. Then I present another model from the acupuncture tradition – the five phases – and demonstrate its depth and refinement as applied to a very difficult patient case. Finally, I offer you my vision of changes that would help this country embrace and benefit from the wisdom of acupuncture.

CHAPTER 12
WHAT CAN ACUPUNCTURE DO BEST?

What *can* acupuncture do best? The practical way to answer this question is to draw from the experiences of successful practitioners. As you read accounts of real patients in earlier chapters, you learned about some of the problems I commonly see in my own acupuncture practice. These represent the range of health issues that most physician acupuncturists manage with acupuncture, alone or by combining it with other therapies.

In Appendix III, I have catalogued one hundred medical problems and offer suggestions for the potential value of acupuncture, based on my review of the medical literature, expert panel conclusions, and my clinical experience. I indicate if acupuncture is likely to serve well as the initial or primary treatment, or if it will be more valuable when combined with other therapies, whether conventional or complementary. This appendix will serve you and your family as a quick reference as to whether you should consider acupuncture for a specific condition.

Favorable published results and expert consensus do not guarantee that acupuncture will work for your medical problem. Results are more strongly linked to your starting condition as a patient, the duration and severity of your problem, and your other ongoing health challenges. Much of acupuncture's value comes from individualizing treatments for each patient. By this I mean that not everyone who shares a similar western diagnosis has the same constitution or carries the same medical history. Therefore, a standardized acupuncture approach to the diagnosed problem might not address other important issues in your health profile.

The three main categories of problems helped by acupuncture are musculoskeletal pain (for example, low back pain), organic illnesses (like bronchitis), and so-called functional disorders (such as irritable bowel). In these three broad categories, I strongly recommend that acupuncture be used in as early as possible and that other approaches be added later, depending on how successful acupuncture alone proves.

Too many physicians and patients consider acupuncture only as the last resort, after all other approaches have failed to bring relief. That is not the most productive use of its potential. In many cases, acupuncture should be the first treatment.

Musculoskeletal Pain

In North America and Europe, the main call for acupuncture services is musculoskeletal pain. Thanks to generous and favorable media coverage and, of course, generally positive results, most people are comfortable with the idea of seeking acupuncture treatments for pain. Pain from muscle stiffness and spasm occurs commonly in Vision/Action people (Chapter 5), and muscle aches and pains accompany the bony deterioration seen later in life in Will/Spirit people (Chapter 7).

Acute pain problems – bruises, spasm, sprains and strains, pinched nerves – are common occurrences in active people of all constitutional compositions, and they can resolve quickly with acupuncture. You can safely use acupuncture as the first and only treatment for uncomplicated muscle and ligament pain, as long as there are no open wounds or broken bones. For example, repetitive strain disorders (carpal tunnel syndrome, tennis elbow, plantar fasciitis, and the like) can resolve with acupuncture alone if treated soon after their appearance. So can other muscular pain patterns—temporomandibular joint pain, muscle tension headaches, upper back and neck muscle pain.

My usual recommendation is to follow a course of a half-dozen acupuncture treatments for new pain problems or pain problems recently turned chronic. I expect to see some change – even if minor – no later than the third or fourth treatment and to know how far acupuncture can change the problem by the sixth visit. If acupuncture makes no difference at all after five or six treatments, then I consider referring the patient for additional treatment modalities that complement the acupuncture.

Acupuncture can be especially helpful immediately *following surgical procedures*, to modify the experience of pain and help with the respiratory and bowel difficulties that sometimes occur. It continues to be useful to ameliorate pain and help return of function during the rehabilitation period following surgery, whether orthopedic surgery (for example, disk decompression, hip replacement, or limb amputation), internal (for example, appendectomy or coronary artery bypass), or surface (for example, lumpectomy or mastectomy).

Chronic pain problems can also be improved or resolved with acupuncture. As a rule, the longer you have had a problem, the longer a course of treatment and the more likely you will need to incorporate additional treatment approaches. If you have osteoarthritis of the knee or shoulder, acupuncture can often give you enough relief that you need little or no medication. If you have muscle and bone pain from degenerative disk disease in the spine, or persistent pain following surgery for a slipped disk or pinched nerve, acupuncture with electrical stimulation can be the mainstay of your rehabilitation.

My approach to a new patient with low back pain, whether or not there is pain running down the leg, is to work initially with acupuncture and electrical stimulation alone for three or four visits to see how much response I can get. Commonly I recommend intermittent or ongoing use of over-the-counter pain relievers or anti-inflammatory medicines to help temper the pain as we progress with the work. If we haven't been able to sustain an improved level of comfort (notice here I say comfort, not necessarily total relief of pain), I'll inject the major muscle trigger points with a local anesthetic in addition to my acupuncture treatments. And I'll recommend the patient consult my physical therapist for additional treatments and exercise training.

A wonderful aspect of acupuncture therapy is its adaptability to the changing requirements of a patient's condition, and its adaptability when combined with other treatments. For example, if your chronic musculoskeletal pain problem is not making good progress after a half-dozen sessions of acupuncture plus electricity plus trigger point injections, finding a physical therapist skilled in manual therapy (deep muscle and connective tissue massage and manipulation) might be just what you need to make the treatments hold. The physical therapist can design specific stretching and strengthening exercises for you to do at home to prolong the effect of the treatments. You might also need to work with a physician trained in osteopathic manipulation techniques, which offer a broad range of subtle and gross movements and adjustments to your bones and muscles. This approach is especially effective with acupuncture therapy.

Acupuncture can be useful for other chronic pain problems, such as post-herpetic neuralgia, peripheral neuropathies, and headaches from muscle tension or other causes. I have been surprised how chronic headaches – even migraines – that have been around for years can respond well to acupuncture. I have also been surprised how common and straightforward problems that I've treated successfully many times in some patients do not improve with acupuncture in other patients. My working dictum is: If it makes clinical sense to treat it, it's worth a try to see what happens.

How many treatments will it take to get as much change as possible in a pain problem? I can only answer this question on an individual basis, after several sessions of acupuncture. In a chronic pain problem, the first half-dozen treatments explore the changes that can be accomplished with acupuncture. I schedule these treatments once or twice weekly until they have an enduring effect. When the discomfort and limitations reach a new and better plateau, the treatments can be separated to every two, three, and, ultimately, four weeks. It might take a dozen treatments to get to once-a-month sessions. Some pain patients can then return as needed if the pain recurs. Others will need ongoing maintenance acupuncture sessions every month, six weeks, or three months. My goal is to see someone as infrequently as possible to maintain the improvements.

Acupuncture treatments limited to the trunk and extremities are less likely to benefit *difficult neurological cases* – spinal cord injury, strokes, and degenerative processes such as multiple sclerosis and Parkinsonism. I have, however, had rewarding responses to a special technique called

Chinese scalp acupuncture, which involves putting needles under the scalp overlying the zone of the brain that is responsible for the problem. Not all acupuncturists are trained in this technique, however; you will need to ask about the doctor's expertise.

Organ Problems

We also call these internal medicine problems, because an internist or other specialist is usually involved in making the diagnosis and managing the care for chronic organ-based problems. Here, again, the adaptability of acupuncture works in favor of the patient. Even if acupuncture is one of several approaches used concurrently, if you start it early you will benefit by having the symptoms resolve more quickly, and you will build up your resilience against them coming back. The four divisions of internal medicine that respond best to acupuncture are the:

- respiratory,
- gastrointestinal,
- gynecologic, and
- genitourinary systems.

Notice here that the first three of these systems involve the Nurture/Duty biopsychotype, and the genitourinary system involves the organs linked with Will/Spirit.

If you are bothered with *chronic or recurrent bronchitis or sinusitis*, acupuncture can help clear the symptoms while restoring the energetic strength of the lungs. The nasal, sinus, and lung symptoms of allergies can also be helped, but I have not found acupuncture alone to be sufficient to permanently modify the immune response in allergic patients. In many cases, just clearing the symptoms and reducing their intensity provides welcome relief, and a few treatments each year during the allergy season is all that is needed.

Common *digestive system disturbances* can also respond to acupuncture. Gastric reflux, gastritis, the pain of stomach ulcers, irritable bowel symptoms, diarrhea, and hemorrhoids can all be relieved with a course of acupuncture treatments. Because most people seek over-the-counter or prescription pharmaceutical treatments for these common problems before finding a physician who does acupuncture, I typically work in collaboration with the medications, aiming to alleviate the symptoms and reduce or eliminate the need for ongoing medication.

In the field of *gynecology*, I have found acupuncture to be especially useful following childbirth for women who don't regain their vitality after the exhaustion of labor and the demands of early maternity. Or a few years later for women who experience ongoing fatigue, often accompanied by chronic low back pain. Acupuncture can likewise be useful in relieving premenstrual irritability and menstrual cramping, as well as in correcting irregular periods.

Acupuncture can help women with fertility problems to regulate their periods, build up the energy of Kidney, Spleen, and Liver to conceive and carry a pregnancy, and overcome the psychological challenges of going through infertility medications and in vitro fertilization (IVF) cycles. Finally, acupuncture can help to stabilize the hormonal fluctuations of menopause. For most of these women's health issues, adding Chinese herbal formulas can reinforce and prolong the effects of needling. On the other hand, I have not found that uterine fibroid tumors, whether symptomatic or not, respond to acupuncture as the primary intervention. Rather, acupuncture can help women prepare for fibroid surgery and recover from it.

Male and female *genitourinary problems* often respond to acupuncture. It's definitely worth trying for the pain and passage of kidney stones, prostatitis, the discomfort of genital herpes, recurrent bladder infections, and irritable bladder. I have witnessed satisfying acupuncture-induced improvements in the bowel and bladder functions following prostate cancer surgery and irradiation. Male and female libido and sexual dysfunction issues usually fit into patterns that can be interpreted and helped in an acupuncture context. Chinese herbs can also assist with these problems.

As with chronic musculoskeletal problems, the more complex and longstanding an internal medicine problem is, the longer the course of acupuncture treatment necessary to achieve a full response. A physician practicing acupuncture will also pursue conventional diagnostic techniques and medical interventions for difficult problems. Medications that are appropriate for symptom control do not interfere with the acupuncture response. In contrast to symptomatic medications, however, acupuncture seeks to bolster the vitality of the patient in order to undo, as far as possible, both the symptoms and the underlying causes of the symptoms.

As with women's health problems, I find that using Chinese herbs can reinforce what I'm trying to accomplish with acupuncture when treating chronic organ problems. The herbal formulas provoke changes in the organ metabolism so that the energetic input from the needle patterns can work deeper and longer. Adding herbs when treating chronic problems can also reduce the need for frequent acupuncture treatments. Not all physicians trained in acupuncture use Chinese herbs, since it is another discipline that must be studied. If this is the case with your doctor, ask him for a referral to an herbalist whose work he knows and respects, and arrange that they work together on your problem.

I have not found acupuncture to be of substantial value as the sole therapy in treating severe and *chronic inflammatory disorders*. Among these problems are ulcerative colitis, rheumatoid arthritis, and autoimmune diseases, especially if the condition has advanced to the stage where it requires strong medications such as steroids or immune suppressants. I do find acupuncture helpful in managing some of the symptoms and in increasing the vitality and resilience of patients with these problems. For me, it's a matter of being clear with the patient regarding what can be accomplished with the needles. For many patients, just feeling better in general is worth the investment. Patients with *cancer* can legitimately consider acupuncture to help with energy, digestion, sleep, pain, and the unpleasant effects of chemotherapy and radiation. The cancer process itself is not influenced by acupuncture, favorably or unfavorably. But with both chronic inflammatory disorders and cancer, Chinese herbs can provide additional symptomatic benefit.

Functional Problems

I don't like this term because, in medical usage, it is often equated with "It's all in your head." From the perspective of medical acupuncture, there is little separation between mind (that is, psychology, emotions, personality) and body, between psyche and soma. Trivial disturbances can be the warning signs of a more important medical process. I also don't like the term "psychosomatic" for the same reasons, although I think it is useful to reveal the dynamics of physical symptoms as they are triggered by states of psychoemotional stress and tension.

The three chapters on the biopsychotypes gave you a range of characteristics and early functional symptoms that can be interpreted and treated in a preventive fashion using acupuncture. Taken together, these early problems fall into three main categories:

- fatigue states,
- autonomic nervous system disorders, and
- immune disorders.

I consider these early problems to be the most fertile ground for acupuncture intervention, because it is possible to return a patient to a balanced and healthy state if treatments are started early. Acupuncture relies on the innate wisdom of the body to balance the autonomic and immune regulatory systems. It makes an ideal treatment for a broad range of functional disorders.

Fatigue states can include a general and ill-defined fatigue expressed in terms like "I feel tired all the time" and "My energy is just not what I want it to be." Fatigue also accompanies or creates mild depression, muscular pain and headaches, and diminished sexual interest. *Autonomic nervous system disorders* manifest as insomnia, anxiety, palpitations, muscle aches, and digestive disturbances. The *common immune disorders* I see are recurrent infectious and inflammatory states that occur without obvious evidence of immune deficiency. The short list includes sinusitis, pharyngitis, bronchitis, gastroenteritis, and recurrent viral infections.

I encourage you, as a conscientious person dedicated to taking good care of yourself, to consult with your physician acupuncturist even for what may be considered by your HMO to be minor symptoms and changes, and to request assistance to attain better health and vitality. These subtle symptoms, which are commonly overlooked in a conventional setting, when combined with past medical history and family medical history, can lead your physician to an explanation and possibly an acupuncture intervention. Acupuncture can be helpful even for the common early or acute stages of *emotional disturbances*, such as anxiety, excitability, worry, melancholy, and fearful states.

For early functional and psychosomatic symptoms that do not respond promptly or adequately to acupuncture, I assist the needle treatments with homeopathic remedies or Chinese herbal products. I generally use homeopathic remedies in low-potency form to aid in acute problems and in high-potency form to treat problems driven by a core psychoemotional disturbance. Acupuncture can be helpful to reduce anxiety or help insomnia, but if the underlying agitation or autonomic disturbance is not alleviated, these symptoms will promptly return. A well-chosen high-potency homeopathic remedy can assist in balancing the psychological dynamics behind a somatic problem. Homeopathic prescribing, however, requires thorough and special training. Ask your acupuncture physician to help you with a referral to a homeopath whose work he trusts.

Finally, a specialized form of acupuncture that involves placing needles on the outer ear can be valuable in managing *substance abuse problems* and reducing reliance on prescription pain relievers. This is not a technique used by all physicians practicing acupuncture. Keep in mind that, to be effective, substance abuse treatments need to take place in the context of a multidisciplinary center, not by solo practitioners.

Potential Complications from Acupuncture

Acupuncture is a remarkably safe and forgiving discipline, especially when we compare its complications to those we accept from drugs and regular medical procedures. What can go wrong? When we put a needle into the body, we always face the risk of perforating a capillary, which can result in a deep or superficial bruise. These are unattractive, but not dangerous. It is also possible to needle too deeply and penetrate into the lung. A partially collapsed lung is rarely a dangerous event and is usually managed just with observation. When we consider how many millions of acupuncture treatments are performed daily around the world, the number of lungs that are collapsed in a year is truly miniscule.

What else can go wrong? Patients sometimes get lightheaded or feel like fainting, not from any damage to the blood vessels or brain, but from the psychological impact of the needles. This is called "needle shock." It might happen at the first treatment, maybe the second. And it usually happens to men rather than women. Our motto is, "At the first treatment, watch for fainting in cops, jocks, and military types." These are usually Vision/Action people who hold a lot of energy in their muscles, and a sudden, unexpected relaxation of this energy can create lightheadedness or fainting.

All acupuncture practitioners in the west use sterile needles. Most employ single-use, disposable needles; those that don't, follow approved sterilization procedures for their needles between treatments. There haven't been cases of hepatitis transmission reported in the United States in the last twenty years, and there are no reports of HIV transmission in the world literature. Occasionally a patient will develop a rash from the needle, presumably a reaction to one of the components in the stainless steel. If different needle brands produce the same effect, these patients should not continue with treatment.

A feeling of spaciness, relaxation, or even fatigue can occur after a treatment. This is especially true following the first one or two visits. If this happens to you, it is important for you to sit in the doctor's office until you're clearheaded, oriented, and able to drive safely. Ideally, arrange to have someone drive you home after the first visit, just in case this should happen.

Sometimes a change in your sleep can occur following the first session or two. You may sleep more profoundly, or more fitfully, or feel as if you were watching yourself sleep. These effects are minor and short-lived and are unique to each patient.

You can diminish the risk of complications by being conscientious in your selection of an acupuncturist. National organizations representing physician and nonphysician acupuncturists maintain lists of qualified practitioners on their Internet sites. The main referral sources are listed in Appendix IV. When selecting an acupuncturist, it is critical that you intuitively trust his or her style, judgment, and professionalism. Without this confidence, you may not be able to benefit from all that acupuncture can offer.

In the next chapter you will see how elegant acupuncture can be in explaining and treating complex and difficult problems as I present another model from the tradition of acupuncture: the five phases.

GETTING TO KNOW YOU

Chapter 13
Five Phases In Action:
An Elegant Paradigm

In earlier chapters I have described Qi and its movement throughout the body in the channels of the energy circulation network. This concept provides a useful organizing principle for acupuncture diagnosis and treatment, especially when the condition is fairly straightforward. But life is not always so simple.

For complex medical situations, physician acupuncturists commonly need a more comprehensive and dynamic model to thoroughly interpret a case. And that's where the five phases graph comes in. The circular five phases graph is an early philosophical attempt to

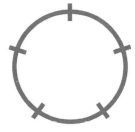

FIVE PHASES

Figure 13.1

describe the visible world and the interaction of its components. It has been in use for more than two thousand years to examine the energetic interactions that promote or relieve disharmony in the body. Beyond that, the five phases graph enables us to understand how seasons, elements, organs, flavors, colors, sounds – the whole range of human experience – influence our everyday physical, emotional, and spiritual health.

Various phenomena and processes can be divided into five dynamically-related organizing groups, represented graphically as five positions equally distributed around a circle (Figure 13.1). How these groups create and control each other can explain the evolution of even the most complex medical disorders – and how to treat them. This exploration will be a little abstract at first. But when we evaluate a patient and explain his medical situation in this model, the value of five phases will become clear.

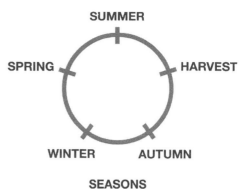

SEASONS

Figure 13.2

One Cycle Generates, Another Controls

Let's start with the *cycle of generation* (sometimes called the "cycle of evolution" or the "cycle of creation"). According to the five phases paradigm, each position on the circle generates, enhances, and supports the position immediately clockwise from it. For example, the seasons (acupuncture recognizes five, not four) can be located around the circle, beginning with spring at the ten o'clock position. In the normal course of time, spring becomes summer (the top of the circle), which leads to harvest (or Indian summer, at the two o'clock position). Harvest turns into autumn (the five o'clock position), which becomes winter (the eight o'clock position), the forerunner of spring (Figure 13.2).

The relationship of the seasons demonstrates the cycle of generation, the intrinsic law of a continual engendering of each position by its

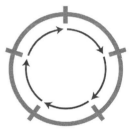

GENERATION CYLE

Figure 13.3

preceding neighbor around the graph. This consecutive movement from position to position reflects the cyclical nature of the day, of the year, and of life. This symbolic relationship among the positions around the circle holds for several dozen sets of factors that can be represented in this model. The relationship serves as a pattern, a law of dynamics, whereby one phase generates the following phase. (Figure 13.3)

A creative cycle of evolution that represents the movement of the sun and the passage of the seasons is easy to comprehend. Some poetic imagination is necessary, however, to appreciate the creative cycle as it applies to the elements. It begins with Wood, which corresponds to spring in the model (Figure 13.4). To say that Wood engenders Fire is

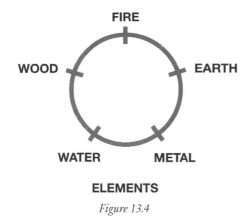

ELEMENTS

Figure 13.4

an acceptable image. Moving in a clockwise direction, Fire creates Earth in the form of the amassed ashes. Earth creating Metal also follows, when one considers that minerals come from deep within the Earth. Metal creating Water is metaphorically problematic: You have to envision water seeping from rocks in the ground to create wells. To complete the cycle of generation, Water creates Wood, in the sense that all living things depend on water to grow.

CONTROL CYCLE

Figure 13.5

Balancing the cycle of generation is a *cycle of control* or "cycle of transformation," in which creation is balanced by destruction, evolution by transformation. Here's the rule that governs the cycle of control: Any given position is controlled by the position that is two places counterclockwise from it on the five phases graph. Thus, Water controls, or keeps in check, Fire; Fire controls Metal; Metal controls Wood; Wood controls Earth; and Earth controls Water. The controlling dynamics connect every other position, creating a star pattern on the inside of the circular graph (Figure 13.5). In the five phases model, each position can generate or control other positions, and each position can be enhanced or diminished in its energetic activity according to the needs of the overall balance.

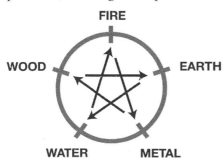

CONTROLLING ELEMENTS

Figure 13.6

The elements attached to the positions (Figure 13.6) lend poetic imagery to the inherent energetic

161

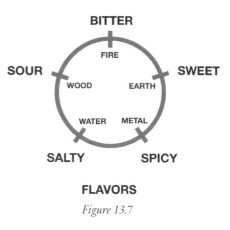

Figure 13.7

dynamics. The Wood position holds Earth in check, just as the forests cover the earth and keep it contained. Earth controls Water, even as river banks and dams keep water contained. Water controls Fire, as water extinguishes fire. Fire controls Metal by melting and forging it into shape. And Metal controls Wood by cutting it with axes and saws.

Five Phases in the Kitchen

The dynamics of this model have many applications in acupuncture medicine. But, rather than moving right away to explore how the five phases graph can be used to sort out complex medical problems, let's first consider how the cycle of control can be used in the kitchen. You might be surprised to discover that abstract acupuncture theory would apply to something so basic as cooking, but in the next few pages you will find a useful application, and a lively experience of the abstract principles. Since each element corresponds to a different category of flavor (Figure 13.7), we can use the flavors to demonstrate the practical reality of the cycle of control.

We all know what it means to overseason a dish, where a flavor exceeds the taste we were aiming for. In five phases interactions, excesses are dampened by stimulating the position that controls them, located two positions counterclockwise on the five phases graph. What follows are a few examples of this law in action. After you have tasted for yourself, you can apply this model to other challenges that involve correcting exaggerated flavors.

Water Dominates Fire: Salt Controls Bitter

It happens, even in these days of designer coffee blends, that a cup of coffee has a bitter taste. The American impulse is to add sugar, and more sugar, and then drink an overly sweetened coffee that still tastes bitter.

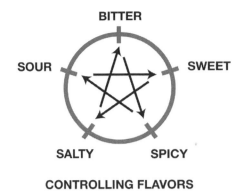

CONTROLLING FLAVORS

Figure 13.8

Try this: Brew of cup of bitter coffee from a notoriously biting blend. Rather than using sugar to modify the taste, crumble a crystal or two of salt into the coffee, stir, and taste again (Figure 13.8). A few small crystals are sufficient to effect the change you want. The goal is not to make the coffee salty, but to use the dynamic influence of the salt to control the bitterness.

There is a lemon tree in our garden in California, and I'm spoiled by having fresh lemons available almost year-round for lemonade or my favorite Brazilian rum drink. Sometimes I am impatient for the lemons to ripen to use in a drink, and I juice them while they still have a green and bitter flavor from picking them too soon (unlike the very sour flavor innate to some lemons). I have saved many noontime picnics and evening gatherings with the pinch-of-salt trick. Try it yourself.

Fire Dominates Metal: Bitter Controls Spicy

Occasionally some of your guests don't like their food as highly seasoned or piquant as you have prepared. You would like to serve them something that they can enjoy, but the hot spices have already been added. You have several choices: you can quickly prepare something different for the sensitive guests; you can dilute the sauce and give more rice to absorb the flavor; or you can take their portion of the dish aside and fix it.

Try this: Crush a few roasted coffee beans, preferably strong, bitter coffee beans, and add them to the sequestered portions (Figure 13.8). Or splash Angostura bitters into the portions while they are still cooking. With either addition, have a neutral party taste the revised food before serving it.

One of my patients had prepared a Mexican mole dish (mole is a sauce containing roasted chili peppers and sweet chocolate, usually served with meat) for a committee dinner meeting, when she was informed too late that most of the committee members were not fond of spicy food. She mentioned this in lighthearted exasperation on her way out of the office, thinking she would get some sympathy from us and then buy a different meal from the delicatessen. Without giving her a lesson on five phases flavor balancing, I told her to add bitter chocolate (not more of the sweetened Mexican chocolate she started with) and five crushed coffee beans to the mole. She called the next day to report that the remedy had worked.

Metal Dominates Wood: Spicy Controls Sour

Sometimes grapefruit juice can be too tart at breakfast, the vinegar too acid for the vinaigrette, or store-bought lemons too sour when juiced for the whiskey sour. Now that you are catching on to the formula, look at the graph and decide what you'd use to right these situations.

That's right. A few drops of Tabasco. It will control the sour and not be detected as a piquant spice in the mix because so little is needed to achieve the result. Please fix the sauces and drinks beyond the watchful eyes of family and friends. Many will not understand or be comfortable with the idea of Tabasco and grapefruit juice at breakfast. But I recommend that you try it.

Wood Dominates Earth: Sour Controls Sweet

This one's easy, and you've probably discovered it for yourself. Take a sip of a cola drink. Very sweet. Now squeeze a wedge of lemon into it. Better balance, not too sweet, and the lemon does not dominate the flavor.

Lemon is probably the best sour agent for drinks. It works in cooking as well; but consider also vinegar or tamarind when you need the controlling effect in a dish that has gotten too sweet during preparation.

Earth Dominates Water: Sweet Controls Salt

This one is obvious as well, but limit your expectations. A dish that has too much salt sometimes simply cannot be corrected. Slightly salty soup, however, is easy to correct with a small amount of sugar. For minor adjustments, refined sugar is usually adequate. I find that a richer sweet flavor such as palm sugar, unrefined cane sugar, or even maple syrup can work more effectively. Again, the challenge is to add just enough to trigger the flavor control without overwhelming the dish with the new flavor.

I married into a family of accomplished cooks, some of them professional chefs. Possessing little intrinsic talent in the kitchen and being overshadowed by professionals and semiprofessionals, I contented myself with preparing drinks and setting the table. Several years ago I went to a series of classes in Thai cooking and developed a zeal for cooking and blending flavors. In the introductory lecture, the instructor explained how Thai dishes are blends of five basic flavors – sour, bitter, sweet, hot, and salty – and that they take their character from the flavor or flavor dynamic that is emphasized within this fundamental matrix. I was delighted to realize that I already knew this perfectly well from my acupuncture training. What she was teaching from her tradition was a living embodiment of the five phases. She was unaware of the formal model of flavor interactions; rather, she knew it intuitively from her childhood training. I felt that I had finally found a small but safe haven in the kitchen, as well as an experimental laboratory for the generating and controlling cycles.

In Thai cooking, sour comes from lime or tamarind, bitter from various herbs and garnishes, sweet from palm sugar, hot from chilies, and salt from fish sauce. Most dishes have a sprinkling of each of these flavors but concentrate on featuring one taste or perhaps the interaction of two tastes. Thus, a soup might have a predominantly hot and sour flavor, and a sauce might feature the interplay between sour and sweet. These two dishes contain a tension between two flavors competing in the controlling cycle.

The creative cycle is featured behind the scenes in the kitchen, and generally the supporting flavor does not get a mention. For example, if the dish is to be predominantly hot and spicy in flavor, it is easy to add so many chilies that the quality and pleasure of the flavor are obliterated by the experience of burning and sweating. Solution: choose only a few of the most flavorful chilies, enough to bring in the spice but very little heat, and add some palm sugar to it while cooking. The sugar, being the supportive flavor, opens and expands the spice of the chili without making it hotter. This is the role of the sweet chocolate in a mole sauce. Try it, and remember you can always tone down excess heat with a splash of Angostura bitters. Another example is using a slosh of fish sauce (a source of salt) to enhance the sour flavor in a vinegar and lime salad dressing.

In the cooking applications of the five phases model, as in the medical applications, the controlling cycle embodies the more dramatic manifestations of interactions and transformations. The cycle of generation continues quietly, consistently helping and nourishing, but drawing little attention.

Medical Applications: The Theoretical Foundation

In daily acupuncture practice, the most practical and comprehensive approach to diagnosis is to categorize clinical information according to the biopsychotypes. We insert needles in patterns to stimulate energy movement through the channel of the most involved organ. Some cases, however, prove to be too complicated to be explained as a malfunction within only one of the biopsychotype subcircuits. This often occurs when problems involve several organs or manifest in unrelated organ systems during different stages of life. The five phases model provides a context in which such complex medical disorders can be organized and interpreted, and treatment can be designed using its two intrinsic relationships: the cycle of generation and the cycle of control.

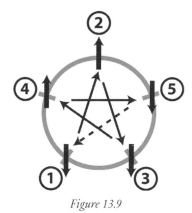

Figure 13.9

The five phases model describes the interactions that occur in the subtle mechanisms of the body to regulate changes and disturbances in any organ. It is a model of functional interactions: the organs along the cycles of generation and control are not linked by tissue or channel connections. The five phases model is a step removed from the network of acupuncture energy circulation; it is not an anatomical or channel chart.

The self-regulating aspect of the five phases graph can be demonstrated in the abstract by tracing a hypothetical deficiency disturbance originating at position 1 in Figure 13.9. Trace the changes step-by-step:

1) Because the energetic deficit at position 1 impedes its control of the activity at position 2, position 2 becomes excessively active.

2) This condition of excess creates an overcontrol by position 2 of position 3, which, in turn, becomes deficient in its energetic reserve.

3) The deficiency at 3 diminishes its controlling interaction with position 4, which, like position 2, becomes excessively active.

4) The excess condition at 4 has a dampening effect on position 5, so that 5 becomes deficient.

5) The deficiency at 5 thus undercontrols position 1, allowing it to return to equilibrium in its energetic presence.

A minor original disturbance normally corrects itself through this five-step balancing process of control cycle dynamics. This energy homeostasis occurs on an ongoing basis within the body. However, when a disturbance is profound or strong or has been present for a prolonged period, the self-correcting effect can fail to create an adequate change, and the disorder becomes a fixed pattern in the patient's energy dynamics. An exaggerated quality can be propagated from any position clockwise along the cycle of generation or starwise along the cycle of control.

Enhancing and nourishing qualities are generally propagated along the generative sequence; pathological or depleting qualities are generally propagated along the control sequence.

Medical Applications: A Case in Point

Let's consider a real patient to see how this all works in the clinical practice of acupuncture. I evaluated this doctor while he was attending a ten-day segment of one of my medical acupuncture training programs. What follows is a narrative of the encounter, including my cataloguing in brackets the information as it was presented.

Dominick Bachowski, fifty-three years old at the date of the interview, is an internal medicine physician who treats patients with severe heart problems or cancer. He presented with the chief complaint of constant fatigue and the inability to build up any muscle mass. He also stated that a gentle game of tennis causes asthmatic wheezing. [Fatigue is too broad a term to link to a specific organ, but ongoing fatigue will most certainly involve diminished vitality in Kidney, and probably other metabolically important organs. Muscle mass is under the supervision of Spleen. (Muscle and ligament movement is under the supervision of Liver, but Spleen influences the flesh itself.) Asthma is linked with Lung and, usually, Kidney. Three organs of potential participation in his disorder are identified within his first few sentences.]

His presenting illness derived from an abrupt and life-threatening case of acute leukemia that was diagnosed five years earlier. He was treated with chemotherapy and then with attempts to induce bone marrow growth. Dom said:

> *I experienced almost every horrible side effect of chemotherapy imaginable. My white blood cell counts were very low because the treatments had actually wiped out my bone marrow. I was so weak that I felt hollow, like a bamboo shoot. I truly felt a loss of essence, and a complete loss of my will to live. I was often near death. My priest anointed me for the last rites so many times I still leave an oil slick when I go swimming.*

The chemotherapy, or a yeast infection while his white cells were not functioning, had created a softball-sized defect inside the tissue of his liver, which caused him severe pain. [Spleen is involved in blood production, and Kidney is the original source of blood and bone marrow. So these two organs show another degree of importance in his problem. Liver is introduced as yet a fourth solid organ to be affected by the disease and treatment process. One of Liver's roles is to store blood, and then supervise its smooth flow.]

During the year of chemotherapy, Dom realized that there were treatments that could complement the conventional approaches to his leukemia. He incorporated diet changes and nutritional supplements, Chinese and American herbs, and guided imagery. His priests and spiritual community helped out with individual and group prayer. During that time his interest in acupuncture was born *"more out of desperation than any belief system or intrinsic open-mindedness."*

By the time he started the medical acupuncture training program, he had already received two years of acupuncture and herbal treatments from a local physician acupuncturist. His white blood counts had more than doubled, the liver pain had abated, and the defect in the liver tissue had repaired itself. But he was still very weak, quite withdrawn, sensitive to noises, and sleeping poorly. [These are general symptoms of a thoroughly depleted vitality, which involves, at its core, Kidney deficiency.] His hearing acuity had diminished during the chemotherapy, and he had lost interest in sexual activity. [These two symptoms are also associated with Kidney energy.] He also listed among his symptoms sinusitis, pain in his lungs with any exertion, spontaneous sweating (especially at night), and a susceptibility to bronchitis at the time of season changes (especially going from Indian summer into autumn or autumn into winter). [These symptoms are all associated with Lung sphere of influence and result from Lung not being able to fulfill its functions.]

Dominick stated that he had occasional heartburn [Stomach Qi not moving downwards], a few varicose veins, and a sensation of heaviness in his legs. [These last two symptoms are linked with the Spleen's responsibility to keep blood within the blood vessels and to hold organs and tissues in place, and thus they emphasize the Spleen's role in his illness.] Finally, he complained of intermittent red eyes and difficulty with his vision while driving at night [Liver again]. He had returned to work, dividing his time between patient care and administration, and incorporating morning and afternoon rest periods into his new schedule.

He revealed so many symptoms that there were only a few remaining areas to explore in his past medical history and review of organ systems. As a child, Dom suffered many sore throats and colds that went to sinusitis or settled into his lungs as bronchitis. [Frequent respiratory infections in childhood suggest that he came into this world with less than an ideal complement of Kidney vitality, or that his early illnesses created an enduring Kidney weakness.] His vision became severely myopic at adolescence [Liver territory]. Even before his leukemia, he suffered from frequent respiratory infections and sinusitis. He was especially susceptible at season changes and during cold weather [Lung and protective energy in general]. At the end of his internship at age twenty-six he contracted viral pneumonia that left him fatigued and wasted [depleted Lung, further depleting Kidney]. He was also found to be anemic at that time and was treated with iron supplements [Spleen, Kidney]. He proceeded straight into his residency and then into practice. Between ages forty and forty-five he experienced another round of fatigue and was first diagnosed with asthma [Lung, Kidney].

Using acupuncture terms, he described his mother as Nurture/Duty, with mixed Metal and Earth features, and his father as Nurture/Duty Earth. He identified his flavor preferences as "sweet first, then spicy, but very close" [Earth and Metal]. His color affinity is black or dark blue: "I always drive a black car" [Water, Kidney]. Dominick is very responsible, has a deep sense of duty to serve as a physician who takes on difficult cases, and participates faithfully in his Polish Catholic religious community. [Metal is his core psychological identity.] He described himself as being a leader in school and his medical community [leadership and drive are Will/Spirit characteristics], but added that there was always an element of fear mixed in his leadership activities [Water, Kidney]. He also acknowledged that he carries anxiety as part of his psychological makeup and that he turns anger inward rather than venting it. He finds church and prayer calming for his anxiety and anger [agitation in Liver-Wood, calmed by increasing Metal].

What was life like before he developed leukemia?

My lifestyle, like most of my contemporaries', was stressful and conducted at a hectic pace. It was manly to work beyond one's limits. I remember making over one hundred forty hospital visits one weekend. Lack of sleep and chronic fatigue are badges of honor. When markedly fatigued, there was always caffeine, sugar, and alcohol to see one through. There was never time for reflection, meditation, or spirituality. That's not what real men did [more evidence of Metal].

By this point, we had a good understanding of Dom's immediate problems, background problems, and constitutional makeup. Still, I was not yet satisfied that I understood why such a catastrophic life event occurred at the time in his life that it did. I asked him what else was going on in his life during the year prior to the leukemia diagnosis, such as increased difficulties at work or home, and other preoccupations or physically or emotionally charged events. Up to this point, he had been composed and matter-of-fact in his replies and explanations. This new question provoked a change in the tone of his voice, which wavered as he spoke.

His cheeks flushed as he explained that during the year prior to his illness he endured his only malpractice suit, and his mother became more strident with her interventions *"to make sure we brought up the children correctly"* [Metal gene pool]. He recalled feeling confident that he could handle these two circumstances, but then his wife's mother began pressuring the family to participate in her commitment to the religious group she had joined. He felt her insistence to be invasive and interfering. He became irritable, even angry, but did not express his feelings to her. His mother-in-law's relentless browbeating created conflict within the family and between him and his wife. His leukemia occurred in the midst of this family dynamic. This was the key I was looking for to understand the pathodynamics of his case.

Dom has a Metal body type—tall, thin, and looking somewhat dry and gaunt, even through his goodwill and positive engagement in the interview process. His pulses and tongue revealed evidence of generalized long-standing deficiency in all the metabolic organs. Our conventional physical evaluation was not especially remarkable: slightly enlarged liver and spleen with tenderness when I pressed over both organs, but not much else, except some eczema on his legs [consistent with frail Lung energy], which was located over the Kidney, Spleen, and Stomach channels. [The location of skin eruption often reflects a disturbance in the organ that is providing the energy for the channel flowing through the rash. In this case, the rash confirmed the weakness in Kidney, Spleen, and Stomach that was identified in the history.]

If I had seen Dom before he was forty years old, I would have quickly identified his Nurture/Duty Metal biopsychotype from his parents' constitutions, the childhood and adult history of recurrent respiratory infections, his Metal body morphology, and his dedication to service and duty. I would have been able to add energy by needling the appropriate organ-energy points on the back, and stimulating them with moxibustion and electricity. This would have treated the background of Kidney deficiency and weak protective energy. To increase the energy in the Lung, I would have activated the Nurture/Duty subcircuit of principal channels with needles in his legs and arms. This needle pattern could also protect him from another episode of anemia, his first overt Spleen symptom. I would also have needled the organ-energy points on the front of the body. Most likely, he would have promptly reported

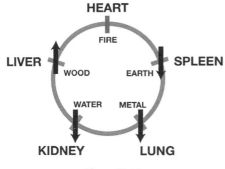

Figure 13.10

feeling more energetic, being more resistant, and having fewer infections. Had he recognized the importance of changing the pace of his life at that time, he probably would have lived out his life with his medical symptoms being contained within the Nurture/Duty subcircuit.

But we were thirteen years and a complicated illness away from that stage in his life. During those years he had continued to tax his core vitality through extreme expressions of his Metal duty and Earth nurturing. Most of his symptoms were still linked to Lung and Spleen, and most recently Stomach. In the interview, however, he revealed more pathology than could be accommodated within the Nurture/Duty subcircuit. He reported Liver symptoms of increased anxiety and irritability, redness in his eyes, and poor night vision. The Liver was vulnerable enough that a hole was burnt in its very tissue. The Kidney deficiency had advanced to a more predominant energetic role with the age forty to forty-five fatigue episode, and, because he pushed himself to work through these symptoms, he burned out Kidney resilience along with a good quantity of essence. Drive and dedication protected Dom from breakdown earlier in his life, but by his late forties, his reserve energy was nearly exhausted.

Dom Bachowski's illness illustrates a disharmony that is too complicated to be explained as an imbalance within the energy subcircuit of only one biopsychotype. His case is an example of five phases in action, and the five phases model serves well to understand his story. Look at the graph of the dynamics that we assembled after the interview (Figure 13.10). This illustration shows the placement of the organs and their correspondence to the elements and other systems. We can immediately place downgoing arrows to represent deficiencies at the positions for Kidney, for Lung, and for Spleen. We also know that something has been going on in Liver: the anxiety and suppressed anger. Even though his entire vitality is depleted, the behavior of Dom's Liver is excessive relative to the underfunctioning of the other three organs. So we place an upgoing arrow at the Liver position.

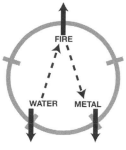

Figure 13.11

Now look at the interactions suggested by the symptom arrows, bearing in mind that serious disturbances are transmitted initially along the control cycle. (Look again at Figure 13.5.) In his childhood Dom had frequent respiratory infections, which were either caused by or caused a Kidney deficiency. Lung (Metal) is only two control steps away from Kidney (Water), via Fire (Figure 13.11). Weakened Water allows increased Fire, (hence the upgoing arrow) thus suppressing Metal (Lung). The early disturbance might have been transmitted in this fashion, then regulated in the Nurture/ Duty subcircuit until further weakening and insult occurred. Dom didn't remember any Fire symptoms from his childhood, adolescence, or early adulthood, but that doesn't negate the dynamics of transmission.

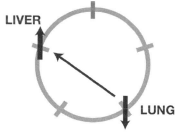

Figure 13.12

There is one control step between Lung and Liver (Figure 13.12). Clearly, Kidney and Lung energies were further weakened during the age forty to forty-five fatigue, which allowed an energetic transmission of the Lung weakness in the form of diminished control on the Liver activities. The undercontrolled agitation of the Liver caused symptoms of irritability and anxiety, which in turn required more of Dom's effort to keep in check.

Enter his mother, the malpractice suit, and his mother-in-law with her religious demands. With his Lung-Liver dynamic already distressed, his psyche absorbed her assault into the Liver sphere. By containing the irritation and anger, the Liver activity increased and exerted excessive control on the position of the Spleen (Figure 13.13). Spleen's functions

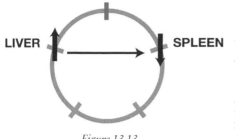

Figure 13.13

were weakened and thereby allowed the leukemia to precipitate. Figure 13.14 summarizes the full energetic pattern. Notice that there is an increasing number of arrows as the whole problem progresses.

Dom's physician-student colleagues and I designed a series of treatments for him that started with a strong boost of Kidney to address the core of his weakness. The second treatment took advantage of the five phases diagnosis and involved energizing the organs that were undercontributing to his system. The third treatment involved back organ-energy point stimulation of Kidney, Lung, and Spleen, followed by an energy-movement stimulation in the Nurture/Duty subcircuit. We gave these treatments to him over the course of ten days, a very large dose of acupuncture in a short time! We then sent him home with recommendations for his acupuncturist to continue with our sequence.

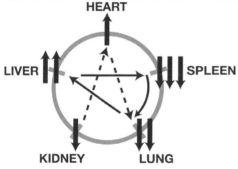

Figure 13.14

The initial follow-up reports from Dom were favorable:

Because of all the attention I had paid to my health between my diagnosis and coming to the acupuncture training course, I had already felt markedly improved. But from a point of view of energy or confidence, I was still far from my old self. With the new treatments, I have felt better than since before my leukemia. My energy has returned. I no longer feel hollow. My sexual interest has returned, and even my hearing is improving. The effect is truly startling. There was also a thirty percent increase in my white blood cell count. Even the microscopic blood exam has returned to nearly normal, with new cells showing normal morphology. This is not supposed to happen following my kind of leukemia.

Most cases are not as complex as Dominick's. Like his own before the leukemia, most patients' histories fit into a single biopsychotype for diagnosis and treatment. But when an illness reaches a certain chronic level, when Kidney and essence have been sufficiently depleted, when additional external forces assault the psyche or soma, an organ can transmit its disturbance outside the containment of its biopsychotype subcircuit. In such cases, the five phases model can be very helpful for understanding the pieces of the puzzle and providing a framework for therapy. Such complex cases truly dramatize the power and beauty of acupuncture.

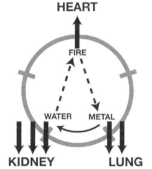

Figure 13.15

Five years later, Dominick had beaten all survival expectations for his illness. To stabilize the good effects of the treatments, he decreased his work load at the hospital and started taking regular afternoon naps. In the sixth year following his diagnosis, however, he accepted the responsibility of medical director for his group, *and* doubled his patient load. For this he paid with increased fatigue, evening fevers, and 3:00 AM wheezing. (Go back to Figure 13.11.) [Kidney's time of greatest energetic activity is from 5:00 to 7:00 PM. Sweating during these hours means his Kidney energy is depleted. Lung's time of greatest energetic activity is from 3:00 to 5:00 AM. Wheezing during this time also suggests Lung energy is depleted.] The wheezing advanced to chronic bronchitis and sinusitis, and a marked increase in fatigue. When recounting this story, Dom shrugged his shoulders and said: *"Being a midwest Polish Catholic internist is a harder addiction to kick than cigarettes and alcohol combined."*

A year later he was diagnosed with prostate cancer (Figure 13.15) Prostate comes under the supervision of Kidney energy. The cancer was successfully removed with surgery, but this left him even more fatigued. "I had to take three weeks off work, and cut back my work load for two months." [Three weeks!] [Two months!!]

Six months after the surgery his wife was diagnosed with breast cancer and, true to his Metal-Duty constitution, he added caring for her without cutting back on his overfull patient and administrative loads. She's doing well, and, so far, the only consequence of this last event has been an increase in Dom's asthma symptoms [Lung] and a craving for summer heat [Kidney is cold from depletion]. I use my best Helmsian baseball-bat psychotherapy on Dom every time I talk with him, bluntly reminding him that few people can survive a second full tour around the control cycle, and that he needs to make substantial and permanent changes in his work habits. For him, it's more important than an emphysematous patient quitting cigarettes, or someone with cirrhosis quitting alcohol.

Five Phases Conclusions

Now that you have observed the essential dynamics of the five phases model, you can better appreciate the sophistication of the theoretical foundations of acupuncture. Even though acupuncture has evolved in a tradition quite different to our own western medical tradition, people are still people, no matter what civilization or era they belong to. The tenets of acupuncture diagnosis and treatment allow physicians trained in acupuncture to use the best of both worlds for the benefit of their patients.

GETTING TO KNOW YOU

CHAPTER 14
IF I WERE CELESTIAL EMPEROR

When I was training in acupuncture I regularly heard my professors preface their comments about a medical or social or political situation with the phrase: "If I were Celestial Emperor…" They used this expression to launch an extemporaneous declaration of their personal opinion of what needed to be done to correct the problem, independent of whether it had anything to do with the topic being discussed or to positions that had been taken just before they addressed the audience. I loved the suppleness of this door opener and asked several of my professors to tell me about the background of the expression.

The image, it seems, is linked to the exalted status of the emperor in classical China. Depending upon who recounted the story, it was either connected to the Han period of early Chinese history (2nd century B.C.) or the Ming period of late Chinese history (16th century A.D.). The emperor in these periods was believed to have a direct connection to heaven, having been appointed by God, and was endowed with clear vision and infallibility regarding matters of his empire. Hence the name "Celestial Emperor." The story further states that the Celestial Emperor, when standing in the center of his Temple of Heaven at noon on summer solstice (the most potent and charged moment of the year, when the sun is at its apex on the longest day), was in direct contact with the wisdom of heaven. When he emerged from the temple, the Celestial Emperor proclaimed to his ministers and subjects his vision for the year. And his divine word was truth and law.

I loved the humor of this conceit and how my teachers used it as a disclaimer to excuse themselves from criticism for violating professorial etiquette. I have tried unsuccessfully to find historical documentation of the story and have asked scholars of Chinese history about its veracity, also without success. Whether the story is apocryphal or not, I, like my professors before me, use it to launch some of my opinions of how the wisdom and practice of acupuncture can best serve our culture and our time.

If I Were Celestial Emperor

- *I would start by improving the general health education and health consciousness of all people.*

A comprehensive model of well-being, illness, and good health practices needs to be part of the basic health education in secondary school, and it needs to be reinforced at home. Obviously, biology class must teach anatomy and physiology, and health class must teach intelligent hygiene and body awareness. But health class can employ the biopsychotype model to help young and curious students understand how people are made up differently. This notion might help put them at ease with their differences one from the other. The biopsychotype model can also provide a context for understanding constitutional strengths and weaknesses and introduce the idea that one's strength is often the route of breakdown.

Further, the recommendations that emerge from the acupuncture model can help young students comprehend and respect their own responsibility for maintaining good health. As they absorb the wisdom of acupuncture, they will get to know themselves more fully and, in the process, appreciate how this knowledge integrates itself into the habits and health care decisions of daily life. Parents should be informed of this new approach to good health through parent-teacher meetings and school-wide presentations.

Beyond the secondary school level, I would expand the training of health educators in hospitals and health maintenance organizations to include the biopsychotype model of constitutional makeup, along with biopsychotype-specific good health recommendations. I would have these institutions offer health education in the form of small group sessions, where the participants can get to know about themselves and ask questions about best health maintenance, as well as the management of illness. The goal in this effort would be to encourage people to become aware of their health imbalances early, before they become fixed and irreversible and, therefore, difficult and expensive to manage. This would be true preventive medicine.

The practical wisdom from the acupuncture tradition can help people understand their combination of qualities, the configuration that makes them unique. This information can provide a roadmap to self-understanding, as well as to recognizing the level of manifestation of early or troubling symptoms. Such an understanding creates a partnership between physician and patient, where the patient can assist by understanding his symptoms and the physician can assist by explaining the options in all matters pertaining to his health care.

- *I would reorganize the learning process in medical school and residency training.*

Currently medical education addresses health and the human organism from a mechanistic perspective, where mind and body are evaluated separately, where the patient is analyzed only objectively, as if his body were a machine. Medical diagnoses are locked into a disease-oriented construct, where outside pathogens are blamed for disturbances almost to the exclusion of the patient's lifestyle or constitution. I would certainly not curtail the advances and applications of new science, technology, and pharmaceutical or surgical interventions, but I would require that a broader perspective be incorporated into the consciousness of medical training.

By this I mean an approach that acknowledges a more humanistic, holistic quality in the lives of both physicians and patients. Such an approach encourages the physician to recognize the connections among spirit, mind, emotions, and body and the interaction of these forces in the generation of illness. It fosters a closer connection between the physician and patient, where the patient is seen in the full context of his life and health. Students and seasoned practitioners alike can benefit from an understanding of healthy states, rather than concentrating uniquely on pathology. Treatment in such a model involves helping the patient to recognize what he can do to heal himself from within, through changes in habits, as well as with interventions from the outside.

How would I accomplish this? I'd start by making sure that medical students appreciate the history of western biomedicine, how Pasteur's germ theory and the evolution of the pharmaceutical industry have shaped what we now consider to be "conventional" and "correct" medicine. It is a fairly short history, when compared to some of the other medical traditions that have existed for a much longer time. They should also understand the historical and contemporary importance of other approaches to health care, such as acupuncture and Chinese herbology, homeopathy, naturopathy, and osteopathy. Just because the American Medical Association does not embrace any of these options does not make them second-class citizens among all the resources to which a physician should appeal while doing his best to help his patient.

I would see to it that acupuncture becomes a standard division of contemporary medicine, no longer marginalized as "alternative" or "complementary." I would shift the paradigm of medical practice to enable acupuncture to become as conventional and widespread as prescribing antibiotics, suturing lacerations, or requesting lab studies. To this end, I would have all medical students undertake a month of intensive acupuncture training in their second year of studies. They would learn the biopsychotypes, the energetic functions of the organs from the acupuncture perspective, and the vocabulary of the elements. I would teach them how to talk to patients as real people, how to touch and palpate them while examining their musculoskeletal problems, and how to insert needles for common pain problems. I would ensure that they understand that techniques like acupuncture can help the body heal itself by activating intrinsic mechanisms of repair and homeostasis.

This way students can begin to understand their patients from the viewpoint of health and imbalance within the biopsychotype paradigm. They can also start early in their training to intervene with a needle pattern – no matter how simple or severe the problem is – at the same time as they are learning the details of physiology and pathology of the organs and the rest of medicine, pharmacology, and surgery. This is the only way a true balance of knowledge and skill will be achieved, a balance that will allow each physician to enter practice fully armed and fully aware of his role, resources, and responsibilities. Obviously, those students and residents who choose specialties where acupuncture is fully integrated will have advanced training and clinical experience before entering practice. And, again obviously, the student acupuncture treatments will be supervised for the correct applications within the full spectrum of conventional medical techniques.

One of the greatest values of medical acupuncture is that it makes sense of early manifestations of disturbances, complaints that are often brushed aside as concerns of the "worried well." The constitutional biopsychotype model contains categories that match both disturbance patterns and acupuncture treatment patterns. This discipline can often explain and affect the difficult-to-pinpoint symptoms in patients.

As part of the expansion and revision in medical education, medical students should also become familiar with the basic diagnostic tenets and clinical applications of other so-called CAM (complementary and alternative medicine) disciplines, in order to best advise and integrate their patients' overall health care. As well-rounded physicians, they will have more than one way of thinking about patients and their complaints.

- *I would redirect clinical research in medical acupuncture to yield genuinely useful information.*

Currently all the research programs investigating the clinical efficacy of acupuncture employ guidelines similar to those used to test new pharmaceutical products. The published articles serve the purpose of calming, reassuring, and placating skeptics in practice, administration, and the insurance industry that there is, indeed, a demonstrable clinical value to acupuncture. While this is a valuable goal in itself, the studies do little or nothing to augment the knowledge base or clinical practice of acupuncture among seasoned practitioners. I call these "I-told-you-so" studies, because any physician experienced in acupuncture already knows through his training and practice that acupuncture has a good chance of a favorable effect in a broad range of conditions.

The biggest problem in these I-told-you-so studies is that their design does not allow for individualizing the treatment for each patient. With drugs, a certain dosage is given to a population having the same diagnosis and meeting a list of inclusion criteria. The drug is usually compared against conventional treatment and/or an inert placebo pill. The results are objectively measured, so far as possible, and the impact of the drug on the illness is evaluated. Problems that receive similar conventional diagnoses, however, can occur in people of quite different constitutions. The acupuncture treatment is aimed at both the problematic symptoms and the constitutional makeup. Although common treatment patterns are used frequently, each treatment is designed specifically for one patient.

As Celestial Emperor I would start with the premise that acupuncture is scientifically real, effective, and safe, and that it can influence most of the symptoms and systems taught in its two thousand-year-long clinical tradition. There are already enough published positive acupuncture studies to move on from the rigid pharmaceutical model of investigation. I would encourage the sort of clinical research that measures changes in more than one symptom, that evaluates general well-being and productivity compared to a pre-acupuncture state, that questions patient satisfaction with the management of their health problems, and that documents the participants' use of other conventional and nonconventional products and services; plus, of course, the change in the symptoms that brought them into the study. These "outcome studies" are a useful approach to evaluate multiple features of change in a large group of patients.

In such studies, different traditions and techniques of acupuncture can be compared, so that serious practitioners can use the results to modify or improve their treatments. Of course, fundamental to such an approach is a body of well-trained and experienced practitioners who can provide creative and responsible treatments. Equally important is that the problems being studied are realistically accessible to acupuncture intervention, that treatment protocols are designed by physicians who have substantial experience treating the problems being studied, and that the recommended needle patterns allow for individualization for each patient.

A shift of this sort in clinical research can create a body of clinical knowledge that will be genuinely useful to patients and practitioners. The favorable results of such studies would also generate a strong impetus for acupuncture to be more fully integrated into medical training and practice.

- *I would revitalize in physicians the confidence to return to being physicians so that patients could re-invest their confidence in the judgment of physicians.*

In this age of medical technology and medical technocrats, the notion of service has been largely discarded from the practice of medicine. This loss is not unique to the profession of medicine; it is ubiquitous in today's society. I remember, for example, when I was a young emperor-in-training, that the concept of a service station was just that, a place where the attendant welcomed the customer and actually provided a service. I could drive to the station and be acknowledged by someone who knew my name or at least recognized me as a regular customer. He'd greet me, fill the tank, clean the windows, check the oil and tires, and take the car into the garage if anything needed attention. Gas station etiquette now means pay in advance, fill your own tank, check your own oil, pay for air if the pumps are working, and interact with preliterate monsters wearing headphones in bulletproof glass kiosks. The concept of service has been lost in the drive for cost efficiency.

Over the past twenty years there has been a parallel devolution in the delivery of health care. The concepts of service, individual attention, caring, and consideration have been largely overlooked in the economic equation of market-driven medicine. The consequences of this trend affect both sides: doctors have become depersonalized as they are forced to work in assembly-line environments under unreasonable time constraints, and patients no longer have confidence that their physicians are making the right medical decisions.

Additionally, an atmosphere of distrust has infiltrated the patient-physician interaction, where the fear of a lawsuit paralyzes physicians and prevents them from offering anything but the strictest protocol-driven interventions. By being unwilling to act on their clinical judgment when treating a patient, physicians generate outrageous expenses for the health care system. Instead of explaining to and engaging their patients in the process of evaluation, they try to protect themselves from criticism or legal assault by ordering every lab test or study that might have a bearing on the case. But much of medical diagnosis and treatment is common sense: only when a case becomes more complex or is unresponsive to common sense treatment should doctors initiate more elaborate evaluations.

In my empire, physicians are once again physicians, doctors who enjoy creative interchange with their patients. Human contact becomes the core of the interaction, and this, in turn, restores the confidence of the patients in suggestions offered by their physicians. In evaluating a medical problem, the physician also understands who the person is that has the problem and appreciates why and how this disturbance came about. Finally, physicians and patients cooperate in preventive measures and consider a variety of options before resorting to pharmaceutical or surgical intervention.

The infrastructure of acupuncture theory and practice can play a major role in this new configuration of health care. The acupuncture interview and treatment bring both the art and science of medicine into play and allow conscientious physicians to practice creatively in at least two disciplines. Physicians trained in acupuncture use this additional discipline not to replace their primary approaches, but to broaden the options available to patients. For them, the line between conventional and nonconventional blurs as they listen more attentively to their patients and appreciate details that they previously overlooked.

Patients, likewise, prepare themselves more responsibly and intelligently for their interaction with their physicians, by understanding as best they can their mix of biopsychotypes and by accepting the responsibility for taking care of themselves. At the same time that they are encouraged to demand complementary services from their physicians, they are expected to educate themselves on good health practices and to undertake revisions in their living habits to encourage better health. Insurance companies and society should not have to pay for personal negligence and indifference to responsibility.

With their additional training, physicians exercise sound clinical judgment and offer their patients integrated options. In this new world, all primary care physicians, including emergency physicians, will be able to execute simple acupuncture treatments for common problems. Even now, I encourage patients to demand that their physicians provide acupuncture treatments (or that at least one physician in the group does acupuncture) for early intervention in musculoskeletal problems, functional symptoms, stress-related manifestations, and fatigue. If the physician determines that a trial of six treatments is safely indicated, start with that, before further tests or a trial of medications. If the changes you hope for don't start to occur, then work with the doctor to continue the evaluation and consider additional therapies concurrent with, or instead of, the acupuncture.

A spirit of creativity rather than formulaic treatment will emerge in the practice of medicine. Physician perception and skill will be used to recognize the unique problems of individual patients. The new creativity in expressing one's physicianship will generate confidence in patients for their physicians and confidence in physicians as physicians.

- *In my empire, acupuncture would be fully incorporated into military medical services.*

Acupuncture is an ideal primary approach for many of the medical problems that arise daily on military bases, such as musculoskelelal trauma, respiratory infections, gastrointestinal disturbances, and headaches. On the frontline of military service, acupuncture can play an important role in managing the challenges of battlefield medical situations, such as anxiety, insomnia, diarrhea, burns, shock, and pain. In the rehabilitation facilities, acupuncture has a valuable role in easing pain from injuries, such as residual limb pain or phantom limb pain that can occur after amputation, and assisting the rehabilitation process in general. In the veterans' facilities, acupuncture can become part of every primary care and physical medicine physician's daily offerings, similar to acupuncture's use in a general civilian population.

I would create a training program in medical acupuncture exclusively for military physicians, so that all bases and military medical environments were generously staffed with qualified physician acupuncturists. Because of the constant turnover of military personnel in the three service branches, a pan-military training program is necessary to continually refresh the physician population with new acupuncturists.

- *I would insist on changes in the policies of health maintenance organizations and insurance companies regarding preventive measures and early intervention with acupuncture and other complementary approaches, along with changes in the attitudes of patients regarding access to these services.*

Health and medical care touch every one of us in a critical center of our lives. As we get to know ourselves, we become vitally aware of how we feel on a day-to-day basis, as well as what we do about what doesn't feel right. We are aware of what we do and don't do about forming healthy life habits. And we carefully pick and choose our professional healthcare assistants as we move through life.

However, how we teach and practice medicine in this country is largely dictated by the medical insurance, pharmaceutical, and medical devices industries, and is policed by the malpractice industry. These four industries are economically and politically very powerful and are unlikely to change voluntarily. While I have been making strong suggestions about finding physicians who offer additional services and who approach medicine with compassion and creativity, I do not want to be irresponsible in suggesting that all their services be guaranteed to have insurance or government reimbursement. There is not a health care system in the world that can afford to sponsor everyone's pursuit of value-added medical modalities.

Governments and insurance plans can barely provide the basics of treatment for the major medical illnesses that threaten quality and duration of life in large sectors of the population. One measure that I would strongly endorse is for the Internal Revenue Service to create tax-deductible incentives for people who invest in legitimate preventive healthcare services. The same concept can apply to insurance companies in the form of lower premiums for members participating in preventive and maintenance activities and services.

Speaking as a realistic emperor, however, I acknowledge that professional services for acupuncture and other complementary modalities are likely to remain partially or totally out-of-pocket expenses for the time being. The advantage is that, while our options and decisions for conventional medical care are in many ways circumscribed by insurance and provider guidelines, what we do with services from practitioners of the complementary and alternative medical disciplines remains our own choice and responsibility.

Taking advantage of acupuncture when it is appropriate in your health situation becomes an issue of quality of life. And quality costs money. We make quality of life decisions daily and annually: schools for the kids, iPODs, Xboxes, DVDs, cars, clothing, food, alcohol, cat food, football tickets, and vacations. If we acknowledge good health as the foundation for making all of life enjoyable and productive, budgeting the time and money for it becomes logical and possible. It's simply a matter of taking the responsibility for your well-being and making the choices to succeed in achievable health goals. It is up to you to accept the responsibility to seek and afford these services.

I strongly oppose – in fact, as Celestial Emperor, I forbid – establishing acupuncture as a service reimbursed by state or federal health care plans, because such plans typically generate an unrealistic universal reimbursement standard, and then lower it, and lower it again, making it difficult or impossible for physicians to provide treatments. I saw this happen in France after acupuncture was embraced by the national insurance system. Over a period of five years the insurers reduced acupuncture reimbursement from a level acceptable for forty-five minutes of physician time, to a level where a physician can now earn more money from a five-minute consultation-and-prescription-renewal visit than he can from even an abbreviated acupuncture treatment. As a consequence, of the thousands of French physicians practicing acupuncture in the 1970s and 80s, fewer than one hundred continue to offer this service today. I'd hate to see this happen in my empire.

The experience of countries with fully socialized medicine systems, such as England, Canada, Australia, and the Scandinavian countries, provides further justification for discouraging governmental reimbursement for acupuncture services. In these countries, physicians and patients alike embrace acupuncture. Because the physicians are given an annual salary based on the number of patients enrolled in their census – and not on how much time they spend with an individual patient – there is no incentive for them to practice a sophisticated level of acupuncture. As a result, they tend to do brief treatments primarily for pain problems, and resort to conventional medical management if they don't see quick results.

I'll indulge in one final patient story, this one about a woman successfully managed for fibromyalgia by a colleague in Switzerland. Living with fibromyalgia is a major and ongoing life challenge for those suffering from it. Thanks to his acupuncture treatments she was able to resume her full-time work responsibilities. Then the national h alth insurance company stopped reimbursing the doctor for his services because he was "spending too much time with each patient," according to their statistics for the average internal medicine doctor. When he argued that reduced drug and laboratory expenses for his patients more than balanced the fees for his additional time, they threatened to force him to return all his insurance-derived income from the previous five years. The national medical association would not defend him, and "advised" him to close his practice. His patient's letter to Geneva's biggest newspaper, two months after her treatments were terminated, summarizes this tragic situation, and serves as a warning to subjects in my empire:

> My daily joint and muscle pains have returned, poisoning my life
> and handicapping me in my profession. I am once again taking
> the same medications that created a stomach problem in the past,
> which itself must now be treated. I work less than half-time, and
> collect government disability payments because of that. The cost
> of my medications each month is more than my doctor's acupunc-
> ture fees were. The insurers might think they are saving money
> when they analyze their columns of numbers, but these savings are
> to the detriment not only of the physicians and patients, but of the
> country's overall healthcare budget.

While I want the government to leave acupuncture reimbursement alone, I would like the private insurance industry to recognize that preventive and early intervention with acupuncture makes good economic sense for the insurers, as well as good health sense for its member-patients. Give physicians the liberty to exercise their judgment without fear of being criticized if they don't do every test and study available before they initiate a trial of acupuncture treatments. Certainly make acupuncture the first therapy in musculoskeletal pain problems, functional problems, and stress-driven problems. You can get five to ten acupuncture treatments from a physician for the price of one MRI or a single epidural steroid injection, and many more than that for the cost of a neurosurgical procedure. If acupuncture alone does not adequately address the problem, then the physician acupuncturist can work with the physical therapist, physiatrist, specialist, or surgeon to continue acupuncture while other measures are undertaken.

This way acupuncture can serve as a modest but practical method of cutting costs for patients, physicians, insurance companies, and hospitals. When physicians comfortably exercise their judgment and make creative decisions, acupuncture can aid both the patient and the economics of the health care system.

In our democratic society, we each have a voice in the design and running of our empire. If you resonate strongly with my vision or several of my positions: Act! Start talking, calling, writing, insisting that you be heard and accommodated. It's only through your will that the spirit of change can evolve and be manifest. Take on the duty to follow through with a small project, such as dealing politely yet firmly with your insurance company, your medical group, or your hospital to encourage them to offer acupuncture through their physicians. These actions nurture change for the benefit of us all.

Acknowledgments

When I started this project I didn't realize how many steps I needed to take between writing a textbook for physicians and a self-improvement book for an intelligent readership. As the manuscript evolved through its many iterations, I have been encouraged and guided by a handful of insightful and helpful critics, whom I would like to honor in this paragraph. Bob Leichtman and Norm Shealy inspired me to rework the spirit of my *Acupuncture Energetics* textbook for a wide audience. Lois Morris recognized the potential in the first draft, and insisted that the focus of the book be the biopsychotype model of self-evaluation. Hal Zina Bennett talked me through reframing the big concepts, David Falkner helped me find my voice for this work, and John Elder drove the creative cataloguing of the material in the appendices. Tom Brosnahan and Joe DiPrisco encouraged me with compliments through each effort and change. I am especially pleased that Glen McKenzie was available to tend to the details of graphics and layout for the book. It was Will Boggs who contributed most to refining the final text. His understanding of the arts of writing, medicine, and medical acupuncture, and of Joe Helms, have resulted in a steady and even flow through the complex material presented in this book. We all thank you, Will.

Of course, many friends and colleagues have read and criticized various chapters during the project. I want to give special thanks to those who went to exceptional extremes in their suggestions: Steve Amoils, Tom DiRenzo, Freda Dreher, Richard Fobes, Mia Fuller, Patty Harvey, Gary Kaplan, Steve Leininger, Anne Rosen, Linda Yemoto, and Rich Zweig. My enduring gratitude goes also to Marty Quan and Emily Ratner, who have been tireless champions of my training programs and of medical acupuncture in the academic environments of UCLA and Stanford. Without their support the professional infrastructure of thousands of American physicians practicing medical acupuncture would not have been possible.

The inspired and disciplined work of Maurice Mussat and Jean-Pierre Muyard allowed me to appreciate the depth and subtlety of medical acupuncture, and to be able to help so many of my patients by applying its principles. The physicians who have taught in the Helms Medical Institute training programs must be recognized for helping reframe the classical acupuncture concepts and integrating them into a contemporary medical environment. I likewise have a profound appreciation for the untiring interest and enthusiasm my students have demonstrated during the last thirty years. Their demands for precise explanations and their generous feedback from their own practices have allowed me to refine and clarify every aspect of this material. I am a teacher because of them. And I am a physician because of my patients. The reports and stories from my patients embody – without exaggeration – the spirit of my practice. They are living confirmation of the value of the integrated approach to medicine.

Finally, I want to thank my wife Pamela, who spent many long mornings tirelessly reading, discussing, and editing with me on the verandah during Nantucket Septembers.

Appendix I

FIVE PHASES

> Chart of Element Associations
> Five Phases Graphs
>> Elements with Creative and Controlling Cycles
>> Organs with Biopsychotypes
>> Flavors with Controlling Cycle

CLASSES OF FOODS

> Cold- and Cool-Producing Foods
> Warmth- and Heat-Producing Foods
> Damp-Producing Foods

BIOPSYCHOTYPES

> Vision/Action Biopsychotype Summary
> Nurture/Duty Biopsychotype Summary
> Will/Spirit Biopsychotype Summary

The biopsychotype summaries contain the salient characteristics and exaggerations for each type. They are intended to serve as an overview and rapid reference. Even though in the chapters some features overlap in two biopsychotypes, in the summaries I have placed the quality or symptom under the organ with which it is most strongly associated. In the "Breakdown" columns, symptoms are listed from top to bottom in general order of severity. In the "Recommendations" columns, all dietary suggestions assume a comprehension of the dictum in the "Eat Well" sections of Chapters 9, 10, and 11: "Most people remain healthy if they eat primarily warming foods cooked fresh and eaten warm; lots of fresh vegetables eaten warm; grains and fiber; a variety of animal protein; moderate amounts of nuts, seeds, and fruits; and few concentrated sweets or fats."

ELEMENT	WOOD	FIRE
ORGANS	Liver Gall Bladder	Master of the Heart Triple Heater (ANS) Heart Small Intestine
GLOBAL QUALITIY	Vision/Action	Action Spirit
SPHERE OF INFLUENCE	Muscles Tendons Nails Eyes	Arteries Pulse Complexion Sense of taste
COLOR AFFINITY	Blue Green Blue-green	Red hues
ASSOCIATED SEASON	Spring	Summer
VULNERABILITY TO	Wind	Heat
FLAVOR ATTRACTION	Sour Citrus	Bitter Roasted
CONTROLS	Earth Sweet	Metal Spicy

EARTH	METAL	WATER
Spleen	Lung	Kidney
Stomach	Large Intestine	Bladder
Nurture	Duty	Will
Digestion	Respiration	Bones
Venous blood	Skin	Joints
Mouth, lips	Excretion	Hair
Touch	Sense of smell	Ears
Yellow	White	Black
Earth tones	All colors	Dark blue
Harvest	Autumn	Winter
Indian Summer		
Dampness	Dryness	Cold
Sweet	Flavorful	Salty
	Spicy	
Water	Wood	Fire
Salty	Sour	Bitter

FIVE PHASES

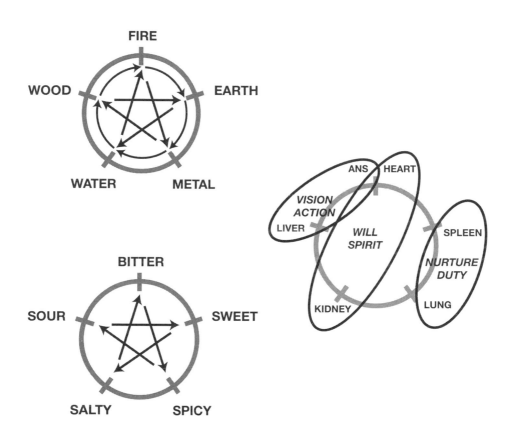

CLASSES OF FOODS

COLD-PRODUCING FOODS

Iced drinks
Iced foods (ice cream, frozen yogurt, chilled milk and juices, smoothies, sodas)
Raw salads (lettuce, celery, cucumbers, tomatoes)
Tofu

COOL-PRODUCING FOODS

Uncooked or processed foods
Uncooked fruits (especially melons)
Uncooked vegetables
Bitter vegetables (endive, kale, chard, spinach)
Fruit and vegetable juices

WARMTH-PRODUCING FOODS

Soups and stews with potatoes, leeks, onions, garlic, rice, oats, lean chicken, turkey, lamb, or beef
Red meat, organ meat
Fish, eggs
Oatmeal, rice
Warming spices (cumin, turmeric, coriander, cardamom, anise, cinnamon, nutmeg, cloves, orange peel)

HEAT-PRODUCING FOODS

Whole milk and dairy products (butter, cream, cheese)
Rich foods
High-fat foods (cookies, pastries, crackers, margarine or vegetable shortening)
Fried foods (hamburgers, fried fast food, French fries, doughnuts)
Refined sugar
Hot spices (black pepper, mustard, chilies, garlic, ginger)
Coffee, black or green tea, alcohol

DAMP-PRODUCING FOODS

Dairy (milk, butter, cream, cheese, yogurt)
Refined wheat (white bread, pasta, muffins, cookies, pies)
Refined sugar (cookies, pies, candy)
Raw vegetables, salads, fruits
Iced drinks and iced foods
Tofu

VISION/ACTION

SPHERE OF INFLUENCE	...IN BEHAVIOR	...IN THE BODY
Liver **Gall Bladder** **(Wood element)**	Liver	Liver / Gall Bladder

Smooth movement of Qi
  and blood through body
	Self-expression and
	  decision-making
	Planning and execution
	  of projects
	Flexibility facing challenges
	Clarity and foresight
		Lateral surfaces of body
		Muscles, tendons, ligaments
		Eyes and vision
		Nails
		Storage and release of
		  circulating blood and fluids
		Resistance to harmful
		  external conditions

Master of the Heart
Triple Heater
(Combined as ANS)
(Fire element)
	Autonomic Nervous
	  System
		Autonomic Nervous
		  System

Energy production and
  movement in internal
  organs: nourishing,
  moistening, warming,
  cooling
Digestion, absorption,
  assimilation, and excretion
	Processing stress and tension
	Fight-or-flight response
	Recover-and-restore
	  response
		Rhythmic beating of heart
		Respiratory and digestive
		  balance
		Internal metabolism,
		  temperature regulation,
		  and homeostasis
		Effect of emotions on body

AS WE ARE MADE UP... (BEHAVIORAL)	AS WE ARE MADE UP... (PHYSICAL)

Vision/Action
Biopsychotype

Warm and spirited — Muscular
Confident things will
  work out — Well-coordinated
    — Good energy
Visual or manual talents — Good vision
Independent — Good nails
Comfortable with planning — Flexible joints
  and decisions — Good digestion
Involved in many projects

Active Expression
Highly motivated
Always on the move
Sports for love of motion
Leader only if necessary

Quiet Expression
Works independently or
  as team player
Creative intellect for
  organizational and
  design projects
Prefers not to be center
  of attention

...SO DO WE BREAK DOWN (BEHAVIORAL)

Stagnant Liver Qi

Anxious, frustrated
Tapping feet or fingers
Clicking pen, doodling
Biting nails
Fiddling with hair
Pacing
Moody
Critical of others
Irritable, or timid
Fondness of caffeine
 and/or alcohol

Plus ANS Imbalance
Sighing
Nervous sweating
Moist palms

Agitated ANS
Jumpy and restless
Overly sensitive to stimuli
Resentful, then angry

Depleted ANS
Fatigue
Everything inside moving
 slowly
Timid, reluctant
Overanalyzing and indecisive

Liver Fire Rising

Undisguised impatience
Extreme anxiety and
 frustration
Bad-tempered and
 grudge-holding
Abuse of caffeine
 and/or alcohol
Dangerous and unpredict-
 able explosions of anger
Aggressive driving

...SO DO WE BREAK DOWN (PHYSICAL)

Predisposed To

Sensitive eyes
Soft fingernails, inflamed
 cuticles
Sensitive to food or
 medications
Sensitive to weather changes
Dizziness
Pain in gallbladder and
 liver area
Difficulty digesting rich
 meals
Liver or gallbladder disease

Stagnant Liver Qi

Muscle stiffness, cramps,
 and contractions
Involuntary twitching in
 arms or legs
Regions of muscle pain
Tension headaches
Jaw tension and pain
Facial tic
Menstrual or fertility
 problems

RECOMMENDATIONS

Plus ANS Imbalance

Vague and variable
  symptoms
Sensitive appetite
Nausea
Abdominal churning
Belching
Migrating abdominal pain
Pounding or racing heart
Insomnia from agitation

Liver Fire Rising

Pain or distention in
  abdomen that rises to chest,
  throat, or head
Red face and eyes with stress
  or anger
Explosive and crippling
  headaches
Trembling in extremities

Know Yourself

Understand and control your
  effect on other people
Explore your behavior
  dynamics through
  journal-writing

Exercise, Relax

Keep the Qi and blood
  flowing
Stretch, walk
Exercise vigorously and
  regularly
Use relaxation or
  meditation techniques

Diet

Moderation keeps the
  Qi flowing
Have biggest meal at midday
Eat fresh greens and sprouts
Avoid rich or fatty meals,
  deep-fried food, high-fat
  foods
Avoid dairy products
Avoid hot and spicy sauces
  and curries
Avoid excessive caffeine or
  alcohol

Seek Treatment

Acupuncture, for acute and
  for maintenance
Manual medicine for
  maintenance
Chinese herbs
Constitutional homeopathy
Anti-anxiety or anti-
  depression medication

NURTURE/DUTY

SPHERE OF INFLUENCE	...IN BEHAVIOR	...IN THE BODY
Spleen (**Earth element**)	Spleen	Spleen / Stomach
Extracting pure Qi from digestive process and sending to Lung	Giving and caring Mental vitality Focus, concentration, memory	Front surface of body Lips and mouth Digestion, from mouth to rectum
Stomach (Earth) **Large Intestine (Metal)**		Maintaining venous blood and lymph in vessels Holding organs in place
Sending energy downward through digestive tract Extracting usable nutrition from digestion and excreting waste		Muscle tone Sense of touch Physical vitality from nourishing energy Menstruation and reproduction
Lung (**Metal element**)	Lung	Lung
Refining pure Qi from air and mixing with Qi from Spleen to create nourishing energy	Order, discipline Regulation Judgment	Respiration Propelling nourishing energy to skin, muscles, organs through principal channels Moving protective energy to surface channels Skin as third lung Body hair Nose, throat, vocal cords Strength of voice Sense of smell

AS WE ARE MADE UP…
(Behavioral)

Nurture/Duty
Biopsychotype

Calm
Orderly
Reliable
Neat

Nurture

Centered, easygoing,
  sympathetic
Generous, compassionate
Tolerant
Good stamina
Likes to touch and be
  touched
Nuclear family very
  important
Good concentration
  and memory
Practical, problem-solving
Enjoys cooking and eating
Bon vivant

Duty

Balanced and reflective
Rational
Organized
Meticulous, precise, reliable
Observant
Follows habit and routine
Matter-of-fact
Loyal
Respectful of the law
Dedicated to good works
Small handwriting

AS WE ARE MADE UP…
(Physical)

Spleen

Rosy complexion
Round, fleshy body
Moist lips
Soothing, melodic voice
Sensitive to flavors and odors
Likes sweet foods
Good digestion
Easy menstrual periods

Lung

Thin build
Slender hands and fingers
Pale complexion
Prefers flavorful foods

...SO DO WE BREAK DOWN (BEHAVIORAL)	...SO DO WE BREAK DOWN (PHYSICAL)	
Nurture	**Spleen**	**Lung**
Over-extended through caregiving	Sour taste in mouth, heartburn, hiccups, nausea	Lowered resistance to viral infections
Over-indulgence in sensual pleasures	Stomach and intestinal gas, bloating, irritation	Allergies
Over-eating	Difficulty losing weight	Acne, dandruff
Introspection, self-absorption	Dissipation and depletion from pursuit of pleasure	Eczema, psoriasis
	Premenstrual syndrome	Dry or wrinkled skin
Duty	Irregular periods	Diminished sense of smell
	Fertility problems	Sinusitis
Overly absorbed in responsibilities	Easy bruising	Bronchitis, pneumonia
Unrealistic perfectionism	Diarrhea, constipation	Asthma, wheezing
Appears detached and unemotional	Dry lips, pale complexion	Emphysema
Bossy and controlling	Weakness and weariness in muscles	**Dampness**
Tendency to melancholy	Anemia	
Risk of depression	Diabetes	Easy weight gain
Attraction to cigarettes		Damp congestion in sinuses, chest, abdomen, or pelvis
		Frequent chest infection with coughing and mucus
		Heavy or long periods
		Fatigue after childbirth
		Varicose veins, hemorrhoids
		Surface capillaries
		Heaviness in legs
		Edema and doughy muscles
		Drooping flesh and organs
		Uterine fibroids

RECOMMENDATIONS

Know Yourself

Nourish your Qi and
  keep it flowing
Be vigilant for over-
  nurturing or self-
  absorption
Learn to say "No"
Relax perfectionist
  expectations
Intercept a melancholy
  mood
Keep a journal to analyze
  and change habits
Control excesses of
  pleasure-seeking

Relax, Exercise

Walking will keep Spleen
  and Lung Qi moving

Eat Well

Moderation
Eat food warm
Relax during meals
Avoid cold- and damp-
  producing foods
Smaller servings, no seconds

Seek Treatment

Acupuncture as early
  intervention
Chinese herbs to reinforce
  acupuncture
Nutritional counseling
Osteopathic manipulation
  of abdominal organs

WILL/SPIRIT

SPHERE OF INFLUENCE	...IN BEHAVIOR	...IN THE BODY
Kidney (Water element)	Kidney	Kidney / Bladder
Activating Qi in all organs	Root of life	Back surface of body
Storing and distributing essence	Will and power	Regulating body temperature and moisture
	Motivation	Essence
	Direction and focus	
Bladder (Water)	Adaptability	Growth and reproduction
Small Intestine (Fire)	Sexual drive	Bones, teeth, joints
		Brain and central nervous system
Digesting, absorbing, and eliminating		Ears and hearing
		Head hair
		Urine production and excretion
Heart (Fire element)	Heart	Heart
Housing the spirit	Vitality, warmth	Heart as arterial pump
Governing blood and vessels	Enthusiasm	Arteries, pulses
	Creativity	Tongue
	Dreaming	Speech and laughter
		Sense of taste
		Sweating

AS WE ARE MADE UP...
(BEHAVIORAL)

Will/Spirit Biopsychotype

Clear-thinking
Motivated, willful
Direct in expression
Hard-working
Balanced as leader or
 follower

Will

Adaptable
Level-headed
Quiet inner strength
Reliable team member
In command of one's life
Forceful when necessary

Spirit

Likes to be seen and heard
Spreads joy and laughter
Talkative, expansive
Bright clothes and jewelry
Seductive
Warm, open
Articulate
Empathetic, intuitive
Thinks, acts, and works
 quickly

AS WE ARE MADE UP...
(PHYSICAL)

Kidney

Warm blooded and energetic
Strong spine and bones
Sensitive to noise and music
Affinity for salty foods

Heart

Clear eyes
Bright and rosy complexion
Very active
Easy sweating

...SO DO WE BREAK DOWN (BEHAVIORAL)

...SO DO WE BREAK DOWN (PHYSICAL)

Will

Spirit

Kidney

Overactive

Imperious attitude

Pushy and competitive

Perceived as arrogant

Depleted

Indecisive

Touchy, doubtful

Insecure, inhibited

Lack of drive and endurance

Easily discouraged

Diminished interest in sex

Overactive

Intense in all behavior

Perceived as frenzied

Dominating, bossy

Quick bursts of anger

Over-confident

Sense of invulnerability

Sexual hyperactivity

Restless, agitated

Distracted

Depleted

Flat personality

Joyless, lacking interest

Profoundly exhausted

Low stamina

Sensitivity to cold

Dark circles or puffy
  under eyes

Premature graying
  or balding

Hearing problems

Balance problems

Generalized pain and fatigue

Cold feet

Joint stiffness and pain

Spine deterioration

Backaches

Kidney stones

Prostate problems

Bladder infections

RECOMMENDATIONS

Heart

Overactive Fire
Sweating
Chest pain
Rapid or pounding heart
Restlessness
Insomnia

Depleted Fire
Physical and mental collapse
Cold feet
Dull complexion
Insomnia
Cardiac problems

Know Yourself

Evaluate your impact on
  other people
Soften your arrogance
Control your impulses
Accept limitations gracefully
Keep your essence warm and
  your spirit moving

Exercise, Relax

Maintain an even pace
Take time for rest and
  recovery
Exercise adequately
Preserve your essence and
  keep the Qi flowing

Eat Well

If Fire, eat cooling foods
Avoid greasy food, avoid
  sugar
If Water, eat warming foods
Steam or wok-fry all
  vegetables
Moderation keeps the
  Qi flowing happily.

Seek Treatment

Acupuncture for
  musculoskeletal, functional,
  and organ disorders
Physical therapy and
  osteopathic manipulations
Chinese herbal formulas
Constitutional homeopathy

APPENDIX II

WHAT'S YOUR CONSTITUTIONAL MAKEUP?

This inventory of characteristics and imbalances contains the questions from Chapter 8, reorganized into broad categories. Scoring each question and tallying the three answer columns will give you a sense of the proportion of each biopsychotype in your constitutional makeup. The first column of scores represents the Vision/Action biopsychotype; the second column the Nurture/Duty biopsychotype; and the third column Will/Spirit.

Try to be honest with your answers, separating what you would like to be from what you really are. There are no "correct" answers. You might also invite your spouse or a close family member or friend to complete the questionnaire on your behalf, and talk about any differences between your perception of you and theirs. It's all part of getting to know you.

Place a 2, 5, or 10 in the score column for each item that represents a quality or disturbance you recognize in yourself, even if it is only approximately accurate in its description. If the item does not seem to apply to you, leave the space blank or place a "0" in it. If one part of a two-part question applies to you, give the full score value for the question.

- "2" indicates that you are familiar with this quality in yourself but that it is not present at all times or a predominant part of your makeup.
- "5" indicates that this quality is present much of the time in your makeup and life activities.
- "10" indicates that the quality is strongly characteristic of who you really are, or that it is a predominant part of your makeup.

When you have tallied each column, I recommend that you read the "Lessons From" chapter for your predominant biopsychotype, then the second in line, and finally the third.

You may download additional copies of this inventory from the book's web site at **www.acupunctureprofessor.com**.

WHAT ARE YOUR STRONG POINTS?

Are you:

good at making decisions and planning things?

usually working on a project, at home and at work?

aware of everything that's going on around you?

limber and well coordinated?

energetic, confident?

usually in good spirits?

pretty good at sports?

well organized and neat?

disciplined?

stable, conscientious, and responsible?

loyal?

nurturing?

reliable and directed?

a good leader, or a good follower?

level-headed? Adaptable?

confident and decisive?

willful?

usually in good health?

intuitive?

Do you:

expect that whatever you set out to do will work out?

know where everything is at your work area, even though it might
    look disorganized to others?

like sports because you like the movement and discipline?

like to cook? Like to eat?

make sure the people with you are having a good time?

page subtotal

216

feel that taking care of your family is the most

    important thing you can do?

get involved in community or religious activities?

get the job done, on time, with the details right?

tend to stick to your routines and habits?

have a tone of voice that sounds as if you know what

    you're talking about?

generally feel happy to be alive?

catch on and learn quickly?

often land in a leadership position?

enjoy playing sports because you like the competition?

try not to let other people see your shortcomings?

play the role of life-of-the-party?

like to wear brightly colored clothing?

sometimes appear intense or speedy to other people?

Have you:

developed your natural visual skills in your professional

    or personal activities?

done a good job organizing your apartment or house; of arranging

    your work area?

Can you:

concentrate and stay focused on what you have to do?

memorize a lot of information?

express exactly what you have in mind to other people?

work hard and keep going for a long time?

quickly sympathize with others or understand their situation?

page subtotal

cumulative subtotal

DO YOU RECOGNIZE ANY EARLY EXAGGERATIONS?

Are your:

muscles stiff, inflamed, painful, or in spasm?

neck, jaw, or head muscles tense?

palms or underarms frequently sweaty, even without activity?

Are you:

anxious, frustrated, or agitated more often than you would like?

constantly working to keep these feelings under control?

aware that if you do not get exercise you will not be able to relax?

locked up inside yourself and too anxious to say anything?

driven to take care of everybody and everything?

too introspective, self-absorbed, or brooding?

feeling as though you haven't felt well since you
gave birth to your child?

easily able to slip into a black cloud or feel sad or melancholy?

self-critical and annoyed with yourself when things
don't go as well as you would like them to?

Do you feel:

that you don't have the energy to get everything done?

that you lack the confidence you once had?

that you keep thinking things over but have trouble
making up your mind?

that your life is busy and successful, but often too stressful?

that you can do outrageous things just because you feel like it?

Do you have worrisome, nervous, or unhealthy habits, such as:

tapping your fingers, pacing, clicking a pen, biting your nails?

page subtotal

cumulative subtotal

drinking alcohol to calm yourself down?

needing coffee, tea, a caffeinated drink, or dark chocolate to keep

going? Or just for the buzz?

drinking coffee (or a caffeinated drink) to make headaches go away?

smoking cigarettes, even though you know it's not good for you?

being too much of a caretaker, getting overly involved in the

lives and problems of other people?

going overboard with the good things in life, eating and

drinking too much?

Do other people see you as:

high-strung or nervous?

timid, reticent to express yourself?

hypochondriacal?

taking a lot of their time telling them your problems?

being too much of a perfectionist?

inflexible in your ideas and decisions?

moving and talking very quickly?

passionate about what you're doing?

arrogant or bossy, when you feel that you simply see how things can

be done correctly sooner than others do?

having a short fuse to your temper, but calming down

quickly, and without grudges?

a good team member, but usually quiet in

meetings and planning sessions?

Do you have:

outbursts of anger when you're irritated with someone, even though

normally you get along well with people?

page subtotal

cumulative subtotal

frequent days when you are short-tempered and irritable?

frequent headaches?

irregular or painful menstrual periods?

soft nails that split or break easily?

the body type that takes on weight easily?

intermittent digestive problems, such as belching, heartburn,
bloating, cramping, or diarrhea?

colds that quickly settle into your lungs or that take a
long time to pass?

recurrent outbreaks on your skin, such as acne or
eczema (as a child or as an adult)?

problems with your back, stiffness in your joints?

intermittent pains in your chest, pounding heart, or
dizzy spells?

cold feet?

Did you:

have frequent bellyaches as a child?

have frequent colds and flu as a child?

start losing your hair or graying in your teens, twenties
or thirties?

ARE YOU LIVING WITH ANY OF THESE IMBALANCES?
When trying to get along with the rest of the world,
do you:

try to avoid being noticed, because you really don't like
to be seen or questioned?

page subtotal

cumulative subtotal

always notice what other people are doing wrong?

remember the people who have crossed you or irritated you?
    For a long time?

need to push your frustration and annoyance deep inside
    so no one sees it?

have trouble making quick decisions or getting things done?

have a hard time apologizing or forgiving?

get angry with other drivers on the road?

neglect taking care of yourself while meeting your responsibilities?

feel obligated to see every project through to the end?

have a personality that frets or worries much the time, about your-
    self, your family, your friends, your colleagues, and the world?

suffer depression to the point of not being able to work effectively?

live with obsessive or compulsive behavior that interferes with your
    daily activities and interactions with your family and friends?

Have you:

had a prolonged period of severe illness or malnutrition in
    your life?

gone through prolonged periods of working too hard and
    exhausting yourself?

had frequent ear, throat, or respiratory infections, or asthma
    as a child?

Are you:

more cautious or fearful than others around you?

becoming more sensitive to noise?

page subtotal

cumulative subtotal

In terms of physical well-being, do you:

have trouble with your eyes or vision?

feel tight and tense somewhere in your muscles almost all the time?

suffer repeatedly from headaches or migraines?

have trouble falling asleep or staying asleep?

feel your heart pounding or beating fast?

have difficulty digesting rich or fatty meals?

experience fullness or pain in the liver area under the right ribcage?

drink too much caffeine for your nerves?

feel heaviness in the chest, abdomen, or pelvis?

suffer chronic phlegmy respiratory problems, such as bronchitis, asthma, or emphysema?

experience pain in the esophagus or stomach, such as acid reflux or stomach ulcers?

have chronic difficulty digesting your food, with bloating, discomfort, constipation, or diarrhea?

experience very irregular periods, or times when your period has disappeared altogether?

have a history of difficulty conceiving or carrying a pregnancy to term?

have uterine fibroids?

feel chronic heaviness or swelling in the legs?

have hemorrhoids or varicose veins?

suffer from prolapsed bladder, uterus, vagina, or rectum?

have diabetes or anemia?

have dark circles or puffiness under your eyes?

page subtotal

cumulative subtotal

often feel chilly inside your body?

have little interest in sexual activity?

suffer regularly from insomnia?

have trouble with your hearing?

have chronic neck or back pain, with or without radiation to arms or legs?

have degenerative or osteoarthritic changes in your spine or joints?

have any urinary tract symptoms, such as kidney stones, frequent bladder infections, prostate problems, difficulty with urination?

have coronary artery or cardiac disease?

WHAT ARE YOUR COLOR AND FLAVOR PREFERENCES?

Do you:

especially like blue, green, or turquoise colors?

especially like yellow, ochre, and earth tones?

especially like red hues?

especially like dark blue and black?

especially like sour, citrus, or acid flavors?

especially like sweet flavors?

like food that has a lot of flavor, even spicy, but not necessarily hot?

want to put extra salt on your food or eat salty snacks?

page subtotal

total

VISION/ACTION NURTURE/DUTY WILL/SPIRIT

YOUR SCORES		
Highest	Middle	Lowest
BIOPSYCHOTYPES IN SCORED ORDER		

Appendix III

Potential Value of Acupuncture
for Common Medical Conditions

In the following chart I have listed one hundred medical conditions for which acupuncture services are commonly sought. This is not an exhaustive list of all medical conditions; rather, it includes problems that are likely to be responsive to acupuncture intervention. I rank each condition with a +++, ++, or +, to give you my clinical sense of acupuncture's potential value in its management. Please remember that all acupuncture responses vary according to the severity and duration of the problem, and the general health of the patient.

- +++ indicates that it is very likely that acupuncture alone will result in a substantial improvement or resolution of the problem;

- ++ suggests that there is a good chance for improvement with acupuncture treatments, alone or in combination with conventional or complementary approaches;

- + means that likelihood is not as good as ++, but that an honest try using acupuncture, in combination with conventional and complementary approaches, is appropriate.

By placing an entry in the "Primary Treatment" column I am stating that it is good medical sense for your physician to start acupuncture treatments for this condition after a initial evaluation and examination, and to use acupuncture as the primary therapy for the problem. This category applies primarily to musculoskeletal pain and common self-limiting medical conditions. I recommend a trial series of up to six visits at a once- to twice-weekly frequency.

A favorable response, even if minor, should begin by the fourth treatment, although in chronic conditions six or eight treatments might be necessary before convincing change occurs. If there is little or no improvement, your physician will decide whether to pursue further studies or referrals, or to add other conventional or complementary therapies.

For those conditions that I identify in the "Complementary Treatment" column it would not make good medical sense to use acupuncture as the primary or exclusive therapy. These problems, however, do have a good chance of responding favorably and promptly to acupuncture, used early in the course of the illness in collaboration with other conventional or nonconventional medical techniques. In chronic conditions acupuncture can provide more thorough relief when combined with other modalities, than can any single modality on its own.

By ranking a condition in both columns, I am suggesting that acupuncture might be of value either as the primary or a complementary treatment, depending on your physician's clinical judgment and the specifics of the case.

In Chapters 9, 10, and 11 of this book I make suggestions from a short list of other time-tested complementary disciplines that enhance the effects of acupuncture for musculoskeletal pain problems, functional disturbances, organ problems, and psychoemotional conditions. Qualified practitioners of these disciplines are widely available throughout the United Sates. It is beyond the scope of this appendix to comment on all emerging alternative and complementary approaches. Please refer to Appendix IV for Internet resources for practitioners.

My short list of complementary disciplines includes:

- *Chinese herbal formulations*;
- *Nutrition*, which can include dietary counseling, supplements, and naturopathic herbal preparations;
- *Homeopathy*, as low-potency remedies for acute problems or high-potency remedies for deep-set or psychoemotional conditions;
- *Manual medicine*, which includes osteopathic medicine techniques of musculoskeletal, visceral, and cranial manipulation, as well as deep-tissue massage;
- *Relaxation techniques*, which can be formal techniques such as biofeedback or autogenic training, meditative or visualization practices, and movement techniques such as stretching and yoga.

Because each patient's condition and constitution is unique, I have not placed these recommendations in a preferred sequence for each problem. Your physician will be able to create a layered treatment program combining acupuncture with approaches that include the standard of care in conventional medicine, and one or several complementary disciplines to give you maximum assistance to overcome or manage your problem. The goals of using acupuncture in an integrated approach are faster resolution of the problem, better pain management, increased energy, improved overall results, and fewer medications and side effects.

CONDITION	PRIMARY TREATMENT	COMPLE-MENTARY TREATMENT	SPECIAL CONSIDERATIONS
Allergies	++	++	
Ankylosing Spondylitis		+	Goals are muscle relaxation and pain relief
Anxiety	+++	++	Acupuncture effective for acute cases, better as complement in chronic cases
Arthralgias / Arthritic Pain	+++	+++	Acupuncture effective in early cases, reduces medication need in chronic cases
Asthma		++	
Balance Problems		++	Chinese scalp acupuncture technique recommended
Bed Sores	+++		
Bell's Palsy	+++		
Breech Presentation	+++		
Bronchitis	+++	++	Effective in acute and chronic cases
Bruises / Soft Tissue Injuries	+++	+++	Effective as primary or complementary treatment
Burns		+++	
Bursitis	+++	++	
Cancer		++	Goal is appetite and energy improvement, pain relief, anxiety reduction, and diminishing side effects of chemotherapy and radiation
Canker Sores	+++		
Carpal Tunnel Syndrome	++		
Cellulitis		++	
Chronic Fatigue Syndrome		++	Acupuncture as one part in multimodality treatment
Chronic Obstructive Pulmonary Disease		+	
Chronic Pain, neurological or musculoskeletal	+++	+++	Acupuncture effective in early cases, reduces medication need in longstanding cases
Common Cold	+++		
Complex Regional Pain Syndrome (RSD)	+	+	Very early intervention gives best results

CONDITION	PRIMARY TREATMENT	COMPLE-MENTARY TREATMENT	SPECIAL CONSIDERATIONS
Constipation	++		
Cystitis, recurrent or chronic		+	
Dental Pain or Procedures	+++	+++	
Depression		+	Acupuncture not appropriate as exclusive treatment
Diabetic Neuropathy		+	
Diarrhea, acute	++	++	
Disc Disease		+++	
Dry Eye / Dry Mouth Syndrome		++	
Dysmenorrhea	+++	++	
Fibromyalgia		++	Commonly requires multiple modalities
Fracture		+++	Acupuncture addresses swelling and pain
Gastritis	++		
Gastroenteritis	++	++	Acupuncture effective for acute cases, better as complement in chronic cases
Gastroesophageal Reflux	++	++	Useful in early and late cases
Gout		++	
Headache, tension	+++		
Hemorrhoids	+++		
Hepatitis		++	Goal is appetite and energy improvement
Herpes Simplex and Zoster, acute	+++	++	Effective as primary or complementary treatment
Hip Pain	++	++	Effectiveness depends on cause of pain
HIV/AIDS		+	Goal is energy improvement and symptom relief
HIV/AIDS Neuropathy		++	
Indigestion	++		
Infertility, male and female		++	
Influenza / Viral Syndrome	+++		
Insomnia	++		
Irritable Bladder	++	+	
Irritable Bowel Syndrome	++	++	
Kidney Stones	+++	+++	
Knee Pain	++	++	Effectiveness depends on cause of pain

CONDITION	PRIMARY TREATMENT	COMPLE-MENTARY TREATMENT	SPECIAL CONSIDERATIONS
Laryngitis	+++	+++	
Low Back Pain	+++		
Lyme Disease		++	Goal is energy improvement
Macular Degeneration		+	Special protocol of ear and hand acupuncture recommended
Meniere's Syndrome		++	Chinese scalp acupuncture technique recommended
Menopausal Symptoms	++	++	
Menstrual Irregularity	++	++	
Migraine Headaches		++	
Mononuleosis		++	Goal is appetite and energy improvement
Motion Sickness	++		
Multiple Sclerosis		+	Chinese scalp acupuncture technique recommended for neurological symptoms, ongoing treatment necessary for neuro and general symptoms
Muscle Aches or Spasm	+++		
Nausea and Vomiting	++	++	
Neck Pain	+++	+++	Effective in acute and chronic cases
Neuritis		++	
Obesity		+	Acupuncture only as part of multidisciplinary program
Osteoarthritis	+++	+++	Goal is pain management and prevention of further deterioration
Parkinson's Disease		+	Chinese scalp acupuncture recommended, on going treatment necessary
Peripheral Vascular Disease		+	
Phantom Limb Pain		++	Chinese scalp acupuncture, ear acupuncture, and body acupuncture recommended
Pharyngitis	++		
Piriformis Syndrome	+++	+++	
Plantar Fasciitis	+++	++	
Pneumonia		++	
Post-herpetic Neuralgia	++	++	Chinese scalp acupuncture technique recommended

CONDITION	PRIMARY TREATMENT	COMPLE-MENTARY TREATMENT	SPECIAL CONSIDERATIONS
Post-operative Pain		+++	
Post-operative Recovery	+++	+++	
Post-partum Recovery	+++		
Post-traumatic Stress Disorder		++	Acupuncture as one part in multidisciplinary program
Premenstrual Syndrome	++		
Prostatitis		++	
Rheumatoid Arthritis		++	
Rhinitis, allergic	+++	+++	
Rotator Cuff Pain	+++	+++	
Sciatica, acute	+++	+++	
Sexual Dysfunction		++	
Sinusitis, acute	+++	++	
Skin Problems, Eczema, Psoriasis	+	+	
Sprains and Strains	+++	+++	
Stroke		++	Chinese scalp acupuncture technique recommended, extended treatment necessary
Substance Abuse, including tobacco and alcohol		++	Ear acupuncture recommended, only as part of a multidisciplinary program
Temporomandibular Joint Syndrome / Bruxism	+++	++	
Tendinitis	+++		
Tennis Elbow	+++		
Tinnitus	++	++	
Torticollis		++	
Ulcerative Colitis / Crohn's Disease		+	
Vertigo		++	Chinese scalp acupuncture technique recommended
Vulvadynia		+	
Whiplash Injury		+++	

GETTING TO KNOW YOU

APPENDIX IV

INTERNET RESOURCES FOR ACUPUNCTURE PUBLICATIONS AND PRACTITIONERS

BASIC SCIENCE AND CLINICAL SCIENCE RESEARCH ARTICLES

Helms Medical Institute
www.hmiacupuncture.com

National Center for Complementary and
   Alternative Medicine
National Institutes of Health
www.nccam.nih.gov/health

American Academy of Medical Acupuncture
www.medicalacupuncture.org

PHYSICIAN PRACTITIONERS

Helms Medical Institute
(physician graduates of HMI programs)
www.hmiacupuncture.com

American Academy of Medical Acupuncture
(physician members of AAMA)
www.medicalacupuncture.org

American Board of Medical Acupuncture
(physicians board certified in medical acupuncture)
www.dabma.org

NONPHYSICIAN PRACTITIONERS

National Certification Commission for Acupuncture
and Oriental Medicine
www.nccaom.org

Acupuncture and Oriental Medicine Alliance
www.aomalliance.org

HOLISITIC MEDICAL PRACTITIONERS

American Holistic Medical Association
www.holisticmedicine.org

OSTEOPATHIC MANIPULATIVE MEDICINE PHYSICIANS

The Cranial Academy
www.cranialacademy.com

American Academy of Osteopathy
www.academyofosteopathy.org

PRACTITIONERS OF HOMEOPATHY

American Institute of Homeopathy
www.homeopathyusa.org

Council for Homeopathic Certification
www.homeopathicdirectory.com

National Center for Homeopathy
www.homeopathic.org